HOW TO BE A HEALTHY VEGETARIAN

The Healthy Vegetarian Guide and Recipe Book

Nancy Addison

Nancy Alisa Gibbons Addison
www.OrganicHealthyLifestyle.com

Limits of Liability and Disclaimer of Warranty

The author and publisher shall not be liable for your misuse of this material. This book is strictly for informational and educational purposes. Nancy Gibbons Addison offers information and opinions, not a substitute for professional medical prevention, diagnosis, or treatment. Please consult with your physician, pharmacist, or healthcare provider before taking any home remedies or supplements, or following any treatment suggested by Nancy Gibbons Addison or by anyone listed in the books, articles, or other information contained here. Only your healthcare provider, personal physician, or pharmacist can provide you with advice on what is safe and effective for your unique needs or diagnose your particular medical history.

Warning – Disclaimer

The purpose of this book is to educate and entertain. The author and/or publisher do not guarantee that anyone following these techniques, suggestions, tips, ideas, or strategies will become successful. The author and/or publisher shall have neither liability nor responsibility to anyone with respect to any loss or damage caused, or alleged to be caused, directly or indirectly by the information contained in this book.

ISBN 978-0-615-39892-1
Library of Congress number: 2011918131

Testimonials

"Nancy Addison knows what she is talking about. When I first started eating vegetarian food, I was hungry all of the time. Then I met Nancy and started eating her delicious food. Nancy's food is really, really, really delicious, and now I feel full and satisfied. I never in a million years thought I would be eating this kind of food and loving it! Going from steak and eggs for breakfast, barbecue pork for lunch, and fried catfish for dinner, with generous helpings of corn, succotash and mashed potatoes with healthy helpings of pie and ice cream, I have embraced Nancy's philosophy of vegetarian food. For me at 80, this sounded like an enormous undertaking and commitment. Within the first week, I could feel the effect of healthy food and healthy living, and am embracing the vegetable world. I have more energy than I ever had and I feel great. She has opened my eyes to a different world. Once you get used to the intricacy of buying, eating, and preparing healthy food, it is really very simple. With her guidance, you start enjoying life with a whole new perspective. After eating Nancy's food for only five days, my blood sugar and my blood pressure were at the most optimum levels, on a consistent basis, for the first time in 16 years. Nancy you are an inspiration to me. Thanks so much for being such a great teacher. I always say: Don't worry, be happy, and feel good. I believe in Nancy so much, that I will even pay you to enjoy her book."

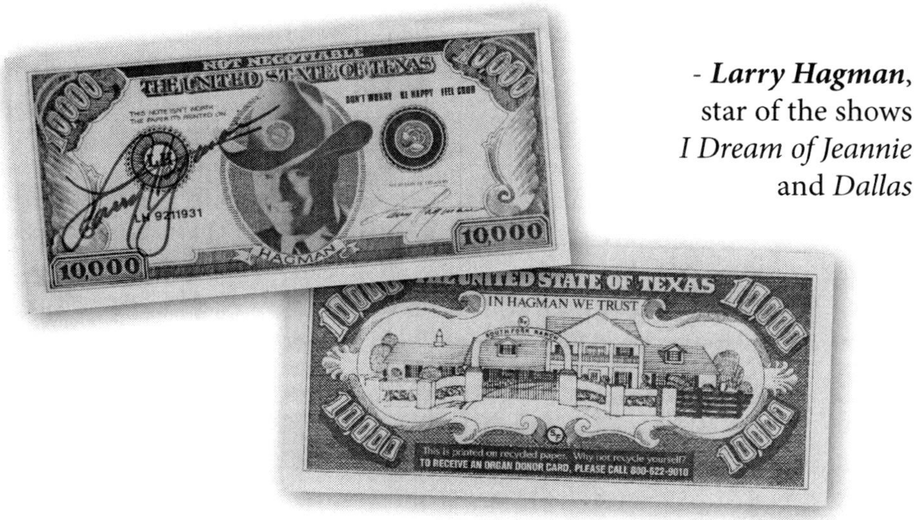

- ***Larry Hagman***,
star of the shows
I Dream of Jeannie
and *Dallas*

"Healthcare trends throughout North America and many parts of the world have struggled for the past several decades in addressing the advancing rates of heart disease, obesity and related illnesses, cancer, and hypertension. The monetary expenditure on these conditions is escalating at rates that neither individuals nor payor agencies are able to sustain. Finally, in Nancy Addison's book *How to Be a Healthy Vegetarian*, both the healthcare provider and layperson have an easy-to-understand resource in reversing the course of preventable disease. Increasing lifespan and quality of daily activities through better decision-making in daily dietary choices is a recipe easily afforded in this time.

"One does not have to look far to see the ravaging effects of chronic inflammation on our health. Peripheral neuropathies, vascular diseases, bowel incompetencies, early cognitive decline, memory disturbances, sleep disorders, hypothyroidism, and a variety of other metabolic/endocrine disorders have all been linked in one form or another to chronic inflammation. Chronic fatigue, pain, and generalized muscle weaknesses are more and more associated with nutritionally deficient diets, sedentary lifestyles, and elevated stress hormones. Nancy now offers an authoritative, well-researched book that is easy to follow and even easier to apply to even the most hectic of lifestyles. Better dietary choices through better understanding and implementation are vital to preventing and reversing today's chronic illnesses.

"Nancy's style and presentation of expert content and topic are inviting and hospitable. You'll want to take in every page and consideration. For both the healthcare provider and layperson alike, reading this book will provide new insights for a long and healthy life for yourself and the lives that you impact!"

- **Michael W. Hall, DC, FIACN**, has been providing chiropractic services for the past 20-plus years. He is a professor of neurology in the clinical sciences department at Parker University in Dallas, Texas. He is an international speaker on the management and prevention of neurological disorders. He is a Fellow of the International Academy of Chiropractic Neurology and a Diplomat of the American Board of Chiropractic Neurology.

Dedication and Acknowledgments

First and foremost, I thank God for the constant love, support, inspiration, knowledge, experiences, and energy that it took to put this book together.

May God bless this book and all who read it.

Heartfelt thanks and dedication to:

Eve Baughman Jung

My last night in Athens, Greece, was a magical night for me, because it started me on a new path of my life's journey. It was Eve's and my last night after studying Mediterranean cooking together on the island of Syros. Thank you so much, Eve, for suggesting that I write this book! Eve, I give you my sincere, heartfelt thanks for your friendship, encouragement, and advice!

and

Amanda Gibbons Addison and Frederick Gibbons Addison

You are the loves of my life. My wonderful children have hung in there with me through thick and thin. You have been my foundation and support over the years as I experimented with food and life in all its venues. You were my original taste-testers! You have helped me prepare, develop, refine, and taste-test all of my new ideas all of your lives. You are my biggest fans, and I am yours. It was you and your friends who provided the inspiration for writing this book, with all the phone calls and e-mails from college, the Peace Corps in Africa, law school, etc. regarding what to buy for your kitchens, for your dinner, and for your health. I compiled a list of information, advice, and recipes to help with the vegetarian lifestyle. I am so very blessed to be able to call myself your mother. My heart overflows with love for you, and I thank you for a lifetime of your unwavering support and love.

Thank you to my wonderful family, especially my mother, Junia Gibbons. I am so thankful for all of your support, generosity, and kindness in my life's journey. You are an amazing family, and I am blessed to be a part of it.

A special thank you to Dr. Gary Massad for contributing the foreword to this book. I am deeply honored by your contribution. I am deeply grateful for your time, effort, faith, generosity, and support. Please know how greatly it is appreciated.

A special thank you to Michael W. Hall, DC, FIACN, for contributing a testimonial review for this book. I am extremely honored that you took the time and energy. Please accept my heartfelt thanks.

A special thank you to Tom Spicer, Suzie Humphreys, Junia Gibbons, Claire Reddick, Amanda Addison, and Gibbons Addison for contributing recipes to this book. Please know how greatly I appreciate it and that I am honored to have them as a part of this book.

Big thank yous to Maryann De Leo, Beth Ann Morgan, and Dr. Gary Massad for the kind testimonials you contributed for my book. I am deeply grateful for the contributions.

An enormous, loved filled thank you from the bottom of my heart to Larry Hagman and Linda Gray for your help, friendship, encouragement, and belief in me.

A big, thank you to Pete Waters and *The Park Cities News*. I have really enjoyed writing columns for your newspaper.

Thank you to Dr. Jan Goss, and Dr. Sharyn Wynters for believing in me. Thank you for your support and continued encouragement.

Thank you to Joshua and the Institute of Integrative Nutrition, the Tree of Life, the Natural Gourmet Institute for Food and Health, Alissa Cohen, and the Australasian College of Health and Science and all of my friends that I met there. I have loved the journey with you.

Thank you to all of my friends and associates at Allie Beth Allman and Associates for all of your kindness, generosity, and encouragement.

A special thank you to my neighbors Randy and Andrea Harrah, Heide and Bob Starr, and Alan Rodriguez and Earl Rector, Nancy Miller and Cindy Williams who are kind, generous, and thoughtful. Thank you for cheering me on my journey and helping me in so many ways.

Julianne Parker, Suann Davis, Susan Williams you have been true and invaluable friends ever since we met. Thank you.

To all of the wonderful friends and neighbors from my life who have honored me with their friendship, never-ending patience, cheerful words of encouragement, and constant support, I thank you all for making my life so much brighter. Bless you all.

I also want to thank my two fabulous photographers, Kelsey Edwards, who took the photograph used on the cover, and Elizabeth Glover, who took the photograph used for the author's picture.

A big thank you to Eugene N. Aleinkoff for being so helpful and generous with your time, expertise, and eff ort that you gave me legally in all of my projects

I also want to thank my ex-husband and the father of my children, who provided years of support and knowledge about health and the environment.

Last but not least, an additional thank you to Jodi Brandon for helping me edit my book, and to my publisher, Donna Kozik, Dina Rocha, and the staff who helped me get it all together. They were amazing and went way beyond the call of duty! I am very grateful for all of your outstanding, hard work and dedication to this project! Thank you; it was an honor to work with you.

I am grateful for all of you. Bless you all. Please accept my deepest heartfelt thanks.

Contents

Author's Note

Becoming a vegetarian, for most, is embarking on unchartered territory!

Adventures in food await! One of the reasons I am writing this book is because many of my friends and my children's friends have tried to become vegetarian, only to find that they were gaining weight eating junk foods or that they just didn't know what was needed to be really healthy as a vegetarian: what to eat, what not to eat, what vegan means, what ovo-lacto-vegetarianism is. In this book, I will guide you through the definitions, the nutritional necessities, the guide to setting up a basic kitchen, what to ask at restaurants, and some basic, delicious recipes that I have developed since I became a vegetarian in 1987. I was a bit bewildered at first with what to eat as a vegetarian and what to feed my children as I raised them as whole-grain, organic vegetarians. Through trial and error and years of research, I found this diet to be easier as time went on and a very healthful way to live. Today there are many more vegetarian choices at grocery stores and at most restaurants than when I was starting out in Dallas, Texas. Things have changed over the years, but there are still many ingredients to be aware of and to be on the lookout for. Reading this book will enable you to be a savvy, healthy vegetarian! You can do this!

Preface

My Life Journey with Food, Health, and Family

Growing up in a large family with five children on a half-acre lot with parents who loved to grow plants of all varieties, cook, and have regular family meals together, it is no wonder that I have found myself an avid gardener and chef. I grow a lot of my own food, and I love to cook for my family and friends. As a small child, I remember trying to help my parents with the garden. Many a Saturday morning were spent weeding parts of the garden or watching my father plant another fruit tree. My parents taught us from the beginning the joy of planting, nurturing, observing, and harvesting our own fruits, vegetables, and flowers. These were always in abundance in our home. My parents spent many hours in the kitchen creating gourmet preserves, dishes, and drinks from the bounty of produce they harvested. Our kitchen was definitely the heart of our home. My siblings and I would help our mother prepare meals. We were also taste-testers for yet one more type of mayonnaise, chutney, sandwich, or dish my father or mother decided to invent that day. A love of cooking, working with the earth, and being creative were given high priority in our lives.

We had a great aunt who loved to give us baby animals for Easter every year. So among our dogs and cats were chickens, ducks, and rabbits. This allowed for fresh eggs now and then, and the animals were also a part of our lives.

My parents dutifully tried to follow the nutritional guidelines our doctors suggested. My mother bought margarine, vegetable shortening, and fortified bread and milk, as well as any other specifics that they said were important for our health and well-being. We had our balanced meals and thought we were doing everything right. My parents were particularly concerned about our eating properly for many reasons, one of which was that when I was 2, my doctor gave me an overdose of penicillin. I was in the hospital and had many blood transfusions and bone marrow tests. My parents were told that I would die before the next morning. Well, miracles do happen, and I survived. (My father always told me that was the night he truly grew to believe in God.)

I survived, but with acute anemia as a result. My mother made me wear a medical alert bracelet on my wrist that said I was allergic to penicillin. She was fearful that I would be in an accident, someone would unknowingly administer penicillin to me, and I would die. Being a skinny, anemic child, I developed an extreme taste for sugar and the energy rush it gave me. It was not unusual for me to have desserts every chance I got. I loved to make sugar and butter sandwiches on soft white bread for an after-school snack. By the time I was in high school, my doctor told my mother that if I wasn't careful, I would end up with diabetes. Well, my mother dug in and really became a watchdog and overseer of everything I put in my mouth. I was given a concerned talk and told exactly what was necessary for me to be healthy. This is when I became aware that sugar was not a healthy choice. I began to see how diet and health are directly connected.

Sweets were kept to a minimum, and my mother made high-protein breakfasts, lunches, and dinners for me. I ate my designated food and avoided diabetes.

College offered a bit of a new food adventure. I tried to stick to my mother's healthy guidelines, but there were times when the Peanut M&M's and the sodas just won out.

During my sophomore year I lived in London and was soon enrolled in classes at Le Cordon Bleu school of culinary arts with my friend. I was in my element. Food was a fun and delicious adventure. Next, Chinese gastronomy was offered at the University of London. What better way to learn than eating gourmet meals for my college class? It was college heaven.

Back in Dallas a few years later, I was married and continuing my fascination with food. Gourmet classes were one of my passions. I attempted to learn everything there is to know about gourmet cuisine. I was driven to learn how to make the best strawberry soufflé in the world. I became the soufflé queen; I made broccoli soufflés, cheese soufflés, chocolate soufflés, strawberry soufflés, and the list goes on.

I began volunteering at the Lighthouse for the Blind. I was working with a group of older individuals who had, because of various circumstances, lost their vision. We were supposed to help them learn the nuances of surviving and thriving without vision. It was hard for some of these people, because they had made their living using their sight, and now they didn't know what to do. They couldn't go for a run or watch TV, and many of them became extremely depressed or suicidal. I am an artist and a certified art teacher in Texas, so I decided to start a pottery class where these folks could socialize and be creative. I played music and taught them how to make simple pieces of art out of clay. I was overdoing it with my hands, though, and soon developed carpal tunnel syndrome. It reached a point where it was excruciating to make a fist or use my hands. I had to take a break from teaching pottery for a while, and I saw doctors about the pain. I had to wear hand splints, and the doctors told me I needed cortisone shots. I got a few of those, and those shots were so painful, though they did bring some relief for a short while. Then the doctors suggested I have surgery. I decided I wasn't going to have the surgery and thought I might try some alternative solutions first. I started to read about carpal tunnel and some natural solutions.

At the same time, I was learning how to make wonderful cappuccinos and lattes. My brother worked at Starbucks and taught me how to use one of those great espresso machines. I was drinking at least two lattes each day. I started to have severe headaches. My doctor asked me how much caffeine I was consuming a day. It surprised me, but I realized I had become a caffeine addict. To deal with this caffeine addiction, I went cold turkey and gave up all caffeine for about three months. I gave it up and then slowly started to allow myself one cup of coffee a day. I didn't think I would ever be able to give up that habit.

Around that time I also began to learn about forms of Omega 3s and how to add these new Omega 3 oils to my diet. I found that when I ate concentrated, nutrient-dense, raw foods on a daily basis and added various forms of "good" oils (including Omega 3s and coconut oil) to my diet, I didn't have the same desire for coffee and caffeine. Eventually my hands started to feel a little bit better as well. I started to think about my diet and how it was affecting my health.

Then one day I found out that I was expecting a baby. We were so thrilled. I was a skinny 100 pounds, and I suddenly found myself ravenous for food. I couldn't stop eating.

My doctor told me that my body was trying to make up for my lack of fat and not to worry about how much I was eating. He also told me that I had hypoglycemia and to eat more often. So I ate and ate and ate. We were blessed with a healthy baby girl, and quickly the urge to eat disappeared. I was still overweight from the birth of my first baby, though, and needed to get back to my regular weight. The doctor told me not to worry about the weight and that it would come off as I breastfed the baby. He also told me that I could not get pregnant while I was breastfeeding. I found out that this was not true: Four months later, I was pregnant again—and still overweight. I was ravenous again, yet trying not to eat all the time. My doctor again told me not to worry and to just eat normally, as long as I took my prenatal vitamins. For the remainder of the pregnancy I ate voraciously once more, unable to control the cravings. I delivered a healthy baby boy, and I was well over 50 pounds overweight. I had never been so overweight; I actually had three chins.

I was determined to lose the weight. I started to take a ballet class a couple nights each week. I felt so self-conscious in my leotard, which was made for pregnant women. I dug in, though, and went faithfully with dreams of being able to wear a smaller leotard. I kept at it and found it was food for my soul. I built my body core back, I obtained a much better posture, I loved the camaraderie, and when I lost myself in the music and the dancing, the rest of the world just melted away. I still take ballet weekly today after 24 years. I may take it forever. It was one of the best things I ever did for myself.

One night, I was reading a long, detailed article in Life magazine about the newest form of corporate farming. It explicitly described the conditions and life of the animals as if they were not living creatures with needs and feelings. It explained the use of drugs and chemicals to make them grow fatter faster and the use of antibiotics to keep them alive, because the conditions in which they were being raised were so horrific that any normal living creature could not survive. (Years later I learned about the environmental destruction and pollution that these types of farms created.) I was absolutely horrified by the information. I put the magazine down, turned to my then-husband, and said, "I can never be a part of this again." At that moment, I became a vegetarian. With two small children under the age of 2 and living in the meat-loving environment of Dallas, Texas, I had a tough road ahead of me. Many of my family members and friends were concerned about my new life choice, yet there I was, deciding to raise the healthiest children I could on a whole-grain, organic, vegetarian diet.

Everyone said that they were afraid my children would be anemic, or that my children would be malnourished, have stunted growth, and be deprived a "normal," healthy childhood. I didn't want to hurt my children in any way, so I started researching everything I could get my hands on to make sure I was doing the right thing for my children and for me. I also realized that I had a family history of heart disease and cancer. I am from Texas and had always lived with the Western and Southern diet rich in meat and fried foods. In fact, a meal wasn't complete—or even a meal—without the big piece of meat in the middle of the plate. The meat was the meal, and everything else was just a side dish. I decided I was going to get healthy, stay healthy, and raise my children to be the healthiest children I possibly could.

In 1987, there were very few places in Dallas where you could buy whole, organic food, much less vegetarian foods. Many of the vegetarian foods tasted terrible and were not made of truly healthful ingredients, so I planted an organic garden, joined an organic seed co-op, ordered food through the mail, and began to make my own whole-food, organic, vegetarian baby food, pasta, corn dogs, breads, and anything else I craved and couldn't find in an organic, whole-grain, vegetarian version. One thing I noticed almost immediately was that I started to eat less food without even trying, I lost weight, and, as if by magic, I no longer had anemia. I had had acute anemia since I was 2 years old. I dutifully had my children's and my blood checked every year for any kind of anemia or deficiency. They were always in optimum health, and my pediatrician said one day that they were the healthiest children he had ever seen. Additionally, and surprisingly, my carpal tunnel syndrome was completely gone.

I was married to an environmental trial lawyer. From all of his cases, EPA reports, and various other research for environmental impact studies, I learned a great deal about the effect the air, water, soil, manufacturing of products, etc. has on our health and our quality of life. I became aware of electromagnetic fields, of types of building materials, where landfills were located, why dry cleaning fluids were toxic and contaminating air and water thousands of miles away, and how all of this and more affects us in everyday life, even if we aren't aware of it. The environment in which we live is critical to our health and well-being. I absorbed this information like a sponge. This gave me added knowledge that the average person does not have.

My children are now out of college. They grow their own herbs, cook their own whole-grain, healthy meals, and find that they are still much healthier than many of their friends. They even have found that they are giving whole-food advice to their friends.

When I first started my vegetarian journey, it was not without challenges. When you start to do something different from what others are doing, they can see this as threatening, because it can make them question what they are doing. Changing the way I was eating and raising my children was so threatening to some people that I was called horrible names at times, and was sometimes not included or invited to certain parties or dinners. Today, so many years later, when so many people are sick with cancer, diabetes, heart disease, high cholesterol, etc., I am feeling good and looking fairly young for my age. Some people are realizing that the idea of eating a whole-grain, vegetarian diet may not be quite as weird as they previously thought. When I have a party, people love to come and see what kind of food I am serving. It is usually all gobbled up quickly, with many folks telling me that it was great. A few of my friends, some of whom were actually ranchers eating an almost all meat and potatoes diet and who simply watched me and listened to me over the years, are now vegetarian and even raw vegans.

I learned so much over the years that I took this knowledge and passion and have become a certified heath counselor, certified raw food chef, and instructor, among other things. I teach others how to grow, prepare, and enjoy fresh, whole, healthy, organic food that can help make their lives healthier and more vibrant. I am excited to share this information with you.

Foreword

by Gary L. Massad, MD

I have been fortunate to practice medicine in many fields and have had the opportunity to study nutrition from some of the best experts in the field. Nancy Gibbons Addison is one of those experts. Nancy promotes thoughtful discussion and improved understanding of disease processes and, most importantly, through *How to Be a Healthy Vegetarian*, she promotes an increased life span for people throughout the world. Food connects us all in some way, shape, or form. We make a powerful choice in what we choose to eat. In this book, Nancy has prepared a menu for health and a prescription for a better, healthier way to do just that.

I've been working with patients and athletes for more than 30 years and have witnessed changes in the approach to nutrition, weight loss, and food in general. Food choices have changed because the composition of food has changed. This book is an invaluable resource that offers a comprehensive overview of protein, carbohydrates, fats, sugars, and vitamins, and includes valuable information about their role in restoring and maintaining your health. Nancy cuts through the myths and hype, and presents the facts as they are. The result is an overview of everything you need to know about living well every day of your life. She makes it easy to understand and even easier to put into action. With the help of this book, you can live longer and get the health results you want.

Nancy is passionate about sharing her knowledge with her loved ones, her family and friends, and, most of all, those who may benefit dramatically by increasing the quality of life through reversing disease. Her knowledge is impressive, and her approach to the selection and preparation of foods is beyond compare. There is always a place for you at her table, so sit back and enjoy the food and feeling healthier.

Gary L. Massad, MD, was head physician at the 1989 World Championships for the United States Cycling Federation in France, attending physician for the United States Cycling Federation (USCF) to the Tour of Texas, attending physician for the Ironman Hawaii, and First National Corporate Medical Director and founder of Occupational Health Centers in America. Additionally, he is attending physician for the United States Triathlon Association, the United States Tae Kwon Do Association, and the United States Cycling Federation.

About Nancy

Nancy is the co-author of *Alive and Cooking: An Easy Guide to Health for You and Your Parents.* Nancy is a certified health counselor by the Institute of Integrative Nutrition and a certified health counselor by Columbia University. Nancy holds a Certificate of Plant-Based Nutrition from eCornell University and the T. Colin Campbell Foundation, and is a board-certified health practitioner with the American Association of Drugless Practitioners. She studied with Natalia Rose and the Rose Program in Detoxification, and is a certified raw food chef, instructor, and teacher with Alissa Cohen. Nancy is certified in Basic Intensive in Health—Supportive Cooking from the Natural Gourmet Institute for Food & Health in New York, nutrition/cooking/food. She is a member of the National Speakers Association, a newspaper columnist, and an author. She has studied at the Mediterranean Cooking School in Syros, Greece, with the Australasian College of Health Science, and conscious farming (organic gardening) at the Tree of Life Rejuvenation Center with John M. Phillips of the Living Earth Training Center. Nancy holds a bachelor of arts degree from Hollins College (now University) in Roanoke, Virginia, holds a lifelong Texas teaching certificate for all grade levels, and is a certified licensed wildlife rehabilitator. She studied at Le Cordon Bleu culinary school in London, England. Nancy also served as secretary of the Earth Society, an affiliate of the United Nations. Nancy is currently studying psychosomatic therapy.

"Vegetarian food leaves a deep impression on our nature. If the whole world adopts vegetarianism, it can change the destiny of humankind."

~ Albert Einstein

Types of Vegetarians

The mainstream vegetarian is the ovo-lacto vegetarian, the broad American version that avoids all animal products that require slaughtering an animal. Ovo-lacto vegetarians eat dairy and eggs. Milk products such as cheeses that don't have rennet in them (rennet is made from the stomach lining of an animal) and non-fertile eggs are allowed. Vegetarian cheeses are made with vegetable rennet, vegetable enzymes, or figs. Ask about ingredients, and find out what kind of rennet is in the cheese you are buying. A lacto-vegetarian only allows milk and milk products in his or her diet.

People who eat chicken and fish are technically not vegetarians, but many call themselves vegetarian. There is frequently confusion about this point. On occasion, I am invited to dinner and served chicken, shrimp, or fish, based on the misconception that a vegetarian eats chicken and seafood. When this happens, simply explain what foods you do or do not eat. In my experience, educating people in a kind and informative manner can make the situation much more positive than acting in a rude or shocked manner. People, I believe, mean well but simply lack the proper knowledge; with the right approach, you can turn the situation around, creating a situation that can accommodate you and be fun for everyone concerned.

Finally, a vegan avoids all products that have an animal origin. A vegan may even avoid honey, because it is made by bees. Many vegans will even go as far as to not use products such as wool, leather, silk, fur, wool, gelatin, lanolin, rennet, whey, casein, beeswax, shellac, carmine, bone, or fat for their bodies or lives. They don't use products that can be made by exploiting a living creature in any way. I believe that a person should see how his or her body and health react to certain foods and lifestyles. I believe it is all about balance. The diet that works for me and my O blood type and lifestyle may not be the perfect diet for someone else.

Try the various vegetarian diet choices that your heart tells you to try, and see how that works. Some people's diet choices may change over time along with age, environment, lifestyle, and circumstance. Balance and flexibility are very helpful and can make life much more enjoyable. I have found that I need to have a little flexibility when I travel to foreign countries, and I don't always have everything exactly as I would like it. Some people I have known who have everything "set in stone" about how they are going to eat or live, run into situations or circumstances that are difficult, and they fall apart when things don't go exactly how they planned. Balance, flexibility, and the ability to live the moment as well you can, can be the difference between success and joy, ***or*** anger, frustration, and/or failure.

Live in the moment, be present, listen to your heart, and try to do the best and right thing for you at the time. Life and our choices are just that: personal choices. I try not to push my way of thinking on others. I do think that one of the best ways to bring about change is from within and by leading my life as I feel is best, so I live as an example of what I believe to be true. I find I bring about more positive change that way. People around me are not faced with a miserable complainer, lecturer, or self-righteous preacher that they want to avoid, but rather a person who lives by what she believes and who brings a little variety to the occasion. Over time, I have learned to deal with food situations in a savvier, more flexible way than I may have when I was younger.

The other day, I was in charge of macaroni and cheese for a dinner, by default. There was some apprehension from the dinner party hostess. I used organic, whole-grain pasta and flour, coconut oil, and some other alternative ingredients that I thought would be healthier. I also used rennet-free, organic cheeses from a farmer I know who raises his animals in a truly cruelty-free way. The cheeses were free of additives like hormones or antibiotics. Everyone loved my mac and cheese!

This was a group that doesn't normally eat this way. In fact, they were all carnivores and didn't really care, or even know, whether the grains were whole or not, or if the milk used was cow's, goat's, almond, rice, oat, organic, cruelty-free, or not. I didn't tell them that the milk I used was made of rice, with no dairy in it at all. I don't think they could even tell. Just by doing this, I may have made a little headway in sharing my vision of a healthier pasta dish.

On another occasion, I made nut cheese for the cheese dish I was asked to bring somewhere. It was received well and with curiosity. I am not sure I converted anyone to my way of eating, but I did enlighten some to the fact that you can make cheese that is actually pretty tasty from nuts.

Find what works for you, and listen to your heart and your own body.

They will tell you the best choices of vegetarian foods for you. You are the best guide and judge of your body and your health. For many of us in transition, with new food choices or life in general, it takes baby steps. Some people will find that eating a little cheese or eggs now and then makes the transition easier. Later, they may be able to cut something completely—or not. Becoming a vegetarian is a journey. Simply start the journey, and see where it takes you!

"Animals are my friends;
I don't eat my friends."

~ George Bernard Shaw

Why Choose Vegetarianism?

The vegetarian diet goes way back in time and was recorded in the sixth century by the Greeks. Today, large numbers of people are switching to a vegetarian diet for health, environmental, and/or ethical reasons. Vegetarians cite many reasons for choosing vegetarianism. One main reason is the idea that the human body was not designed for consuming meat. We don't have the correct teeth for tearing, our saliva isn't as acidic as carnivores', our digestive stomach juices are not acidic or strong enough to digest meat well enough on an ongoing basis, and our intestinal tract is long and curvy, which allows meat to go too slowly through the passage. Because of the long intestinal tract, undigested meat can stay in the intestine too long, allowing it to putrefy and rot in the intestines, and allowing toxins and acid to build up and create inflammation and disease.

Consider these facts:

- According to McGill University, studies show that people on healthy vegetarian diets have "lower risks of coronary artery disease, colon cancer, hypertension, and diabetes and lung cancer."[1]
- In the book *Prevent and Reverse Heart Disease*, Dr. Caldwell B. Esselstyn, Jr., former president of the medical staff at the Cleveland Clinic, says you can reverse heart disease with no drugs and only a plant-based diet: "Based on the groundbreaking results of his 20-year nutritional study—the longest study of its kind ever conducted—this book explains, with irrefutable scientific evidence, how we can end the heart disease epidemic in this country forever by changing what we eat. Dr. Esselstyn convincingly argues that a plant-based, oil-free diet cannot only prevent and stop the progression of heart disease, but also reverse its effects."[2]
- Walter Kempner, MD (1903–1997), founded the Rice Diet. He believed that a diet of rice, fruit, and vegetables did miraculous things for people to gain back their health. According to John McDougall, MD, "He treated hundreds of people at Duke University where he prescribed a diet of rice, vegetables and fruit that reversed hypertension, diabetic funuscopic changes, heart failure

(cardiomegalyard EKG changes), kidney and obesity."[3]

- Dr. T. Colin Campbell, PhD, professor emeritus at Cornell and co-author of *The China Study* (the most comprehensive human nutrition study to date), advocates a plant-based diet on a scientifically based platform for optimum health. Dr. Campbell told his class at Cornell University:

> Plant-based eating is a superior way of eating. Benefits of eating this way: Live longer, look and feel younger, have more energy, lose weight, lower blood cholesterol, prevent and even reverse heart disease, lower your risk of prostate, breast and other cancers, preserve your eyesight in your later years, prevent and treat diabetes, avoid surgery, vastly decrease need for pharmacetical drugs, keep bones strong, avoid impotence, avoid stroke, prevent kidney stones, keep your baby from getting type II diabetes, alleviate constipation, lower your blood pressure, avoid Alzheimer's, beat arthritis and more.[4]

Furthermore, he said about tests he has done where disease started in populations where meat protein was introduced into the diet:

> My early research gave me the understanding that animal protein when tested experimentally was substantially different from plant protein in its ability to promote tumor development. It turned out that animal protein had its effect by operating through a constellation of integrative mechanisms. The division between animal and plant foods was a signpost of a division of the kinds of foods having an effect on cancer.[5]

In this class on plant-based nutrition, I learned of many studies that prove that many people can actually be healthy or overcome illness on a plant-based diet.

Some people choose a vegetarian lifestyle for moral reasons that have nothing to do with health or medical benefits. They simply believe that eating animals is wrong, or they do not want to have anything to do with a living creature's cruel treatment or death.

Many people throughout the ages have chosen to be vegetarian for various reasons, among them: Pythagoras, Aristotle, Plato, Leonardo Da Vinci, Benjamin Franklin, Albert Einstein, Thomas Edison, George Bernard Shaw, Mohandas Gandhi, Paul McCartney, Stella McCartney, Carl Lewis, Hank Aaron, Mike Tyson, Martina Navratilova, Doris Day, Danny DeVito, Alec Baldwin, Joan Baez, Ellen DeGeneres, Larry Hagman, Linda Gray, Michael Bolton, Mary Tyler Moore, Joaquin Phoenix, Dave Scott (six-time Ironman triathlon winner), Brendan Brazier (two-time Canadian 50 K ultra-marathon champion), and the list goes on and on. In this group of great, enlightened minds and/or great talents, there is a common bond. It is a choice.

Professors speak firmly on this subject as well. For instance, Tom Regan, professor emeritus of philosophy at North Carolina State University, says that animals have "inherent value" and "basic moral rights" to "the right to respectful treatment" and "basic moral right not to be harmed."[6] Then there is Gary L. Francione, professor of law at Rutgers School of Law, who argues that animals are sentient: "[A]ll sentient beings should have at least one right—the right not to be treated as property" and there is "no moral justification for using nonhumans for our purposes."[7] Peter Singer is a professor of bioethics at Princeton University. Mr. Singer's argument is that there is "no moral justification" to use animals as food, that "our use of animals for food becomes questionable—especially when animal flesh is a luxury rather than a necessity," and that it's "better to reject altogether the killing of animals for food, unless one must do so to survive."[8]

Environmentally and globally, becoming a vegetarian can save thousands of gallons of water, thousands of gallons of oil, thousands of acres of rainforest, and the list goes on. It is by far the best choice for any positive contribution to the earth and all of its inhabitants for anyone who truly cares about the future of the planet. Over time, I have become acutely aware of the impact a meat-eating diet has on the environment and its resources. A plant-based diet does not drain resources from the earth, or create environmental pollution and damage the same way a meat-based diet does. There are many ways a vegetarian diet can help with the environment, beginning with preserving our precious water supply. Raising livestock requires enormous amounts of water. The Water Education Foundation in Sacramento, California, is a non-profit organization that states that it is "the only impartial organization to develop and implement educational programs leading to a broader understanding of water issues and to resolution of water problems."[9] Their most recent publication, entitled "Water Inputs in California Food Production," references the studies of Herb Schulbach and Jim Oltjen, Gerald Ward, and other sources. Their final analysis concludes that it takes 2,464 gallons of water to produce a pound of California beef.[10]

Marc Reisner, a former staff writer at the Natural Resources Defense Council and the author of the highly acclaimed *Cadillac Desert,* a history of water and the American West, wrote in the *New York Times* in 1989:

> In California, the single biggest consumer of water is not Los Angeles. It is not the oil and chemicals or defense industries. Nor is it the fields of grapes and tomatoes. It is irrigated pasture: grass grown in a near-desert climate for cows. In 1986, irrigated pasture used about 5.3 million acre-feet of water—as much as all 27 million people in the state consumed, including for swimming pools and lawns.... Is California atypical? Only in the sense that agriculture in California, despite all the desert grass and irrigated rice, accounts for proportionately less water use than in most of the other western states. In Colorado, for example, alfalfa to feed cows consumes nearly 30% of all the state's water, much more than the share taken by Denver.... The West's water crisis—and many of its environmental problems as well—can be summed up, implausible as this may seem, in a single word: livestock.[11]

More and more water aquifers and wells are being drained, rivers and lakes struggle to remain clean, and over 40 percent of the water in the United States is being used for irrigating crops to feed livestock.

> Agriculture accounts for 87 percent of all the fresh water consumed each year. Livestock directly use only 1.3 percent of that water. But when the water required for forage and grain production is

> included, livestock's water usage rises dramatically. Every kilogram of beef produced takes 100,000 liters of water."[12]

Farm runoff from these large, concentrated farming areas is creating huge pollution problems with waste that includes antibiotics, hormones, and pesticides. The impact of these types of farms on our environment and our water resources is enormous. A plant-based diet can make a significant impact.

In a *Harper's* magazine article, Richard Manning states:

> Eighty percent of the grain the United States produces goes to livestock. Seventy-eight percent of all of our beef comes from feed lots, where the cattle eat grain, mostly corn and wheat. So do most of our hogs and chickens. The cattle spend their adult lives packed shoulder to shoulder in a space not much bigger than their bodies, up to their knees in shit, being stuffed with grain and a constant stream of antibiotics to prevent the disease this sort of confinement invariably engenders. The manure is rich in nitrogen and once provided a farm's fertilizer. The feedlots, however, are now far removed from farm fields, so it is simply not "efficient" to haul it to cornfields. It is waste. It exhales methane, a global-warming gas. It pollutes streams. It takes thirty-five calories of fossil fuel to make a calorie of beef this way; sixty-eight to make one calorie of pork.[13]

"Cornell University's David Pimentel says that it takes 40 calories of fossil fuel to produce one calorie of protein from feedlot beef, while it takes only two calories of fossil fuel to produce one calorie of protein from tofu—a huge difference in energy expelled for food."[14]

These studies both show that an enormous amount of energy is used to produce meat for consumption. This is an unnecessary waste of energy as well an enormous burden and drain on the earth's resources.

Our earth's natural resources are being destroyed so quickly from the cumulative effect of raising animals for human consumption. The Nature Conservancy states that "every second of every day one football field of rainforest is being destroyed."[15] Much of this forestland is being cut down to farm and raise livestock, which is then exported to the United States and ends up in fast-food hamburgers. According to the Rainforest Action Network, 55 square feet of tropical rainforest are destroyed to make every fast-food hamburger made from rainforest cattle.[16] They say this is an area about the size of a small kitchen.

> It is gone forever each time one of these hamburgers is eaten. It is even worse because with each square foot of rainforest gone, up to 30 different plant species, 100 different insect species and dozens of bird, mammal and reptile species are destroyed. The rainforests are so important because half of the species on earth live in them and the forests are vital to the world's oxygen supply.[17]

Lillie Ogden says in an article in *Vegetarian Times* magazine that factory farms' waste gives off ammonia and methane, in addition to casting off dust and particles into the air. These cause air pollution, acid rain, and respiratory problems. This type of pollution can be seen as a brown type of haze or cloud.

> Since these farms are so large and often use huge manure lagoons the most obvious pollution is the horrible smell, which affects communities nearest the farms. The bad smell is the least of the dangers to the environment.... Methane may be the most serious gas given off from livestock. In fact, the meat industry is the number-one source of methane throughout the world, releasing over 100 million tons a year. Methane is a gas that traps heat in the atmosphere and causes the earth's temperature to rise. Noam Mohr, in his report on global warming, says that "methane is 21 times more powerful a greenhouse gas than carbon dioxide." Theoretically by reducing the amount of meat eaten throughout the world we could slow down methane production and therefore global warming.[18]

"The single most environmentally important choice," according to Lillie Ogden, "is to eat a plant-based diet."[19]

John Robbins has statistics in his book *Diet for a New America,* first published in 1987, that are factual and simply speak for themselves:[20] (Remember that these statistics are over 20 years old.)

- Number of people worldwide who will die as a result of malnutrition this year: ***20 million***

(When I looked up a newer number in May 2011, I found that 925 million people do not have enough to eat—more than the populations of the United States, Canada, and the countries of the European Union combined.[21])

- Number of people who could be adequately fed using land freed if Americans reduced their intake of meat by 10%: ***100 million***
- Percentage of oats grown in the United States eaten by livestock: ***95***
- Percentage of protein wasted by cycling grain through livestock: ***90***
- Increased risk of breast cancer for women who eat meat daily compared to less than once a week: ***3.8 times***
- Number of US medical schools: ***125***
- Number of US medical schools requiring a course in nutrition: ***30***
- Nutrition training received by average US physicians during four years in medical school: ***2.5 hours***
- Most common cause of death in the United States: ***heart attack***
- How frequently a heart attack kills in the US: ***every 45 seconds***
- Average US man's risk of death from heart attack: ***50 percent***
- Risk of average US man who eats no meat: ***15 percent***
- Risk of average US man who eats no meat, dairy, or eggs: ***4 percent***
- Amount of water used in production of the average cow: ***sufficient to float a destroyer***
- Gallons of water needed to produce a pound of wheat: ***25***
- Years the world's known oil reserves would last if every human ate a meat-centered diet: ***13***
- Years they would last if human beings no longer ate meat: ***260***

- Percentage of all raw materials (base products of farming, forestry, and mining, including fossil fuels) consumed by United States that is devoted to the production of livestock: ***33***
- Percentage of all raw materials consumed by the United States needed to produce a complete vegetarian diet: ***2***
- Percentage of US antibiotics fed to livestock: ***55***
- Percentage of staphylococci infections resistant to penicillin in 1960: ***13***
- Percentage resistant in 1988: ***91***
- Response of European Economic Community to routine feeding of antibiotics to livestock: ***ban***
- Response of US meat and pharmaceutical industries to routine feeding of antibiotics to livestock: ***full and complete support***
- Common belief: ***The US Department of Agriculture protects our health through meat inspection.***
- Reality: ***Fewer than 1 out of every 250,000 slaughtered animals is tested for toxic chemical residues.***
- Number of animals killed for meat per hour in the United States: ***660,000***

Regardless of the reason for choosing vegetarianism, being extremely healthy on a diet with no meat (any living creature) or even animal products is easy. Being a vegetarian is a little bit of a learning challenge at first, and it takes some planning and a little knowledge, but it is extremely rewarding and gets easier and easier.

Vegetarians are making a huge difference in the world in many ways. You are in good company.

"I do feel that spiritual progress does demand at some stage that we should cease to kill our fellow creatures for the satisfaction of our bodily wants."

~ Gandhi

Part I

Basic Guidelines for a Healthy Vegetarian Lifestyle

Listed in alphabetical order and not in order of importance.

I cannot tell you how many people I meet who tell me they used to be vegetarian, but they had to go back to eating meat because they just weren't healthy or getting enough food. This makes me very sad. I know there are a few things that are vital for health on a vegetarian diet, but it is really easy, if you just know what to take and where to get it. Eating high-quality food is important for any diet. The body becomes much cleaner and more vibrant if it is getting the best variety of nutrients. The body becomes more aware of problems. Taste buds are cleaner and more discerning.

What we eat becomes our blood and our cells, so I recommend buying organic whenever possible. If we eat foods that have poisons on them or put into them by genetically modified seed, then we are ingesting poison. Avoid any foods that are processed, so you aren't ingesting MSG, potassium bromate, chemicals, and other additives that the FDA allows to be put into food. Many people just need to add some nutrient-dense, concentrated food to their diet in order to feel satisfied on a deep cellular level. This may be because soils have become depleted and food just isn't as nutrient-dense as it was a hundred years ago. Studies have shown a decrease of anywhere from 40 to 80 percent in nutrients in the food today as compared to food in 1914.[22,23]

Eating living, fresh food can feed the body on a more deep cellular level, in comparison to cooked foods. I have learned to eat more raw, living, fresh foods. I add more living concentrated foods to my diet. Everyone should eat nutrient-dense foods, with more minerals, and fermented probiotics-rich foods. A combination of all of these things can help immensely.

Top Priorities for Vegetarians

1. Consume only whole grains when eating anything made from grain (like pasta, bread, crackers, and chips), and avoid corn and wheat (especially genetically modified varieties). If you would like to lose weight, definitely cut out corn and wheat. Gluten-free grains are preferable.
2. Consume no sugar or as little sugar as possible. Do not use fake sugar substitutes in any way, shape, or form. Stevia, dates, and raw, organic honey are my top choices for sweeteners.
3. Make sure you are getting enough protein each day and that your diet contains a variety of proteins, so you get the right amino acid complex combinations.
4. Consume only good fats. Make sure you get enough of the essential fatty acid Omega 3 in particular.
5. Make sure all of the B vitamins, especially B12, are in your diet and absorbed well.
6. Make certain that you are not low in any nutrients. Iodine, iron, calcium, zinc, Vitamin D, and magnesium are all important nutrients and should not be overlooked.
7. Make living and whole foods a major part of your diet. Chew food thoroughly, and try not to water down the digestive enzymes when eating.

Calcium

Calcium is an important mineral. Calcium is necessary for maintaining bone strength as well as for muscles to move and for nerves to carry messages between the brain and other parts of the body. "In addition, calcium is used to help blood vessels move blood throughout the body and to help release hormones and enzymes that affect almost every function in the human body."[24]

The body will pull calcium from the bones in order to regulate the pH balance of the body. Meat is very acidic and can upset the body's pH balance. "Animal proteins can inhibit the absorption of calcium," as reported by McGill University.[25] Vegetarian food that is not processed is primarily very alkalizing and helps maintain a good pH balance. Because of this, vegetarians may not need as much calcium as carnivores. Good sources of calcium are broccoli, kale, collard greens, and mustard greens, as well as fortified tofu or soy milk. Magnesium helps with the absorption of calcium.

Cleanse, Cleanse, Cleanse!

There are many reasons to cleanse and clean out the inside of the body on a regular basis. Clean cells and a clean body, inside and out, are the secrets to having more energy, looking younger, and having a stronger immune system.

The reason we *need* to cleanse is that we acquire toxins in our bodies on a regular basis. Our bodies become acidic through stress and the foods we eat. These toxins and acids hurt our bodies deep in our cells. How can the body have a clean liver, blood, or lymphatic system if it is filled with toxins, acid, and waste? Key factors of a truly healthful system are having a clean intestinal system and having frequent, high-quality, and thorough bowel movements.

We absorb most of our nutrients though the intestinal wall. If it is clean, we are able to absorb them; if it is not, and is instead full of waste and rancid debris, then the body won't get the nutrients it needs because of the blockage. Dr. Anthony Bassler, a gastroenterologist, said, "Every physician should realize that the intestinal toxemias (poisons) are the most important primary and contributing causes of many disorders and the diseases of the body."[26]

We live in a world that is quite literally saturated with toxins. We can get toxins by breathing in polluted air, taking showers in chlorinated tap water, drinking tap water, and eating foods when we don't know their source or preparation method—the list is endless. We also live in a society that has a high level of acid as a biproduct of stress and the foods we eat. Apparently the concept of balancing acid in the body has been around since the 1930s, when Dr. William Howard Hay published a book called *A New Health Era* in which he proclaimed that all disease was caused by an accumulation of acid in the body. In a more recent book, *Alkalize or Die,* Dr. Theodore A. Baroody, ND, DC, PhD, says essentially the same thing: "The countless names of illnesses do not really matter. What does matter is that they all come from the same root cause...*too much tissue acid waste in the body!* [author's emphasis]"[27]

You can buy pH strips at most health food stores to check your body's pH. "If your saliva stays between 6.5 and 7.5 all day, your body is functioning within a healthy range. The best time to test your pH is about one hour before a meal and two hours after a meal. Test your pH two days a week."[28]

Your body's pH balance is critical to survival and health. It is as important as body temperature. Our bodies love us and will try to protect us from toxins by placing fat around them so they won't hurt us. The more acid and toxins we have, the more fat cells our body will make. If we can eliminate these acids and toxins, we give our body no reason to create or hang on to additional fat.

> The over-acidification of the body set in motion a destructive cycle of imbalance, overweight, and disease.... Too much acid in the body robs the blood of oxygen, and without oxygen the metabolism slows. Foods digest more slowly, inducing weight gain and sluggishness, and, worse still, causing the food to ferment (rot!). Fermentation creates yeast, fungus and mold throughout the body. These are all living organisms, so they need to "eat" and when they overgrown in an acidic body they feed on your nutrients, reducing the chemical and mechanical absorption of everything you eat by as much as 50 percent.[29]

"Mild acidosis can cause such problems as:

- Cardiovascular damage, including the constriction of blood vessels and the reduction of oxygen.
- Weight gain, obesity and diabetes.
- Bladder and kidney conditions, including kidney stones.
- Immune deficiency.
- Acceleration of free radical damage, possibly contributing to cancerous mutations.
- Hormone concerns.
- Premature aging.
- Osteoporosis; weak, brittle bones, hip fractures and bone spurs.
- Joint pain, aching muscles and lactic acid buildup.
- Low energy and chronic fatigue.
- Slow digestion and elimination.

- Yeast/fungal overgrowth."[30]

I recommend doing a cleanse that will detoxify the body and adjust the pH balance of the body for a minimum of three days and as long as 21 days. (I do a month-long cleanse every January in order to start off the new year fresh and renewed after too much holiday and party munching.) I recommend doing a cleanse on a regular basis, a few times a week, year-round. This will keep the inner environment of the body's digestive system cleaner, healthier, and able to support a healthy immune system.

Another reason for cleansing is that our intestines can get thick with plaque over time. This "mucoid" plaque can be left from consuming foods like milk, wheat, and meat. This mucoid plaque can be thick and rubbery, and can even look a little like a rope when it finally exits the body.

In the book *Tissue Cleansing Through Bowel Management*, Dr. Bernard Jensen, DC, ND, PhD, addresses this:

> The heavy mucus coating in the colon thickens and becomes a host of putrefaction. The blood capillaries to the colon begin to pick up the toxins, poisons and noxious debris as it seeps through the bowel wall. All tissues and organs of the body are now taking on toxic substances. Here is the beginning of true autointoxication on a physiological level. One autopsy revealed a colon to be 9 inches in diameter with a passage through it no larger than a pencil. The rest was caked up layer upon layer of encrusted fecal material. This accumulation can have the consistency of truck tire rubber. It's that hard and black. Another autopsy revealed a stagnant colon to weigh in at an incredible 40 pounds.[31]

Dr. Richard Anderson, ND, NMD, addresses the subject of plaque as well. Dr. Anderson has written two books on cleansing: *Cleanse and Purify Thyself Volumes 1 & 2*. His expert experience with colon cleansing conveys much of this in his two books. In an article on colon plaque, he says:

> The phrase, 'mucoid plaque,' is a coined term

> that I use to describe various conditions found throughout the body, especially in hollow organs and the alimentary canal. It is a substance that the body naturally creates under unnatural conditions, such as attack from acids, drugs, heavy metals, and toxic chemicals.[32]

Professional cleanses, like colonics or enemas, can get this old, left-over waste and plaque out of the intestinal tract as well. Along with this comes an additional benefit: A major part of the body's happiness chemical, serotonin, is synthesized in the gastric-intestinal tract. No wonder people feel happier and better when their bowels are clean, functioning well, and in the optimum way!

Garden of Life makes a nice, easy cleanse, but for those who wish to create their own cleanse, here are a few different types of cleanses that I have used and found to be very effective.

High-Fiber Cleanse

This is a basic cleanse that I have been doing for over 25 years and raised my children on. It is a good, basic fiber and chlorophyll powder combination. The two things that I think are most lacking in the American diet are good, healthy fiber and good, healthy green foods. This cleanse has both. It is, quite simply, the ingredients of good, healthy food that most people lack in their normal, everyday diet. The nutrients will feed your body as well as help flush and pull toxins and acids out of the cells, then the fiber will absorb these toxins as well as expand out like a sponge. When you drink a lot of water, this will create a cleaning effect of dragging out with the sponge-like fiber the particles, plaque, and other debris that might be lodged in the intestines. Each time you do a cleanse, it will clean out a little more. Think of the layers of an onion. When you start you will get one layer, and the next time you get the next layer. Do this morning, noon, and night for three to 14 days or more. You will have to make a personal decision about the length of your cleanse. Many physicians think 21 days is the best length for a cleanse. You may want to consult your physician before starting a cleanse, and you may want to do a cleanse under the guidance of your physician. Many wonderful physicians and clinics have juice fasts, cleanses, and other programs that you can do under the guidance of their doctors. (I have some listed in the Resources.)

Each time you do a cleanse, it will get easier. Eventually, or maybe very quickly, you will see a difference in how you feel. You may eventually find this is a very good part of your daily or weekly regime. If you have trouble drinking green, powdery, fiber-y drinks, buy the green concentrated powder and the psyllium husks in a capsule form. You can buy these ingredients at most health food stores or grocery stores.

Note: This is my favorite cleanse, but this cleanse is only for someone who is able to have regular bowel movements. If you are not having regular bowel movements, then you may need to simply consume raw, fresh vegetable juice on a regular, three-times-per-day, daily basis, or do colonics, until your bowel movements are regular.

This cleanse calls for a kalenite pill. "Kalenite is a blend of eight herbs known for their ability to support proper elimination through the colon, liver, kidneys and lymphatic system, as well as helping to tone these organs of elimination so they can function more efficiently."[33]

I actually do this cleanse a few times a week, year-round, as a normal part of my diet. When it is possible, I consume fresh, organic green barley grass or wheat grass juice instead of the powdered or liquid concentrate form of green food. Fresh is always best, but the concentrated, powdered form makes it easy to use anytime and anywhere.

Ingredients:

1 kalenite pill (pulls toxins from your cells naturally and helps you not feel queasy)

1 tsp. concentrated raw organic green food powder (in capsules or powder form; freshly juiced greens would be the most optimum, but this is the next best choice)

1 tsp. organic psyllium husks

½ tsp. freshly ground, fresh, organic, raw pumpkin seeds (optional, but pumpkin seeds work really well with parasites)

1 tsp. raw, organic chia seeds (chia seeds add the anti inflammatory, essential amino 3 fatty acids).

1 probiotic capsule

1 digestive enzyme

Directions:

1. For one to three full days, do only the green juice or powder and

chia seeds. This would consist of eight to 10 capsules, one heaping teaspoon of raw, organic green food powder, or a 6- to 8-ounce glass of freshly juiced organic greens with no additives and the 1 teaspoon chia seeds, three to four times a day. Start first thing in the morning. Drink an 8-ounce glass of mineral-rich water, coconut water, or freshly juiced greens or ginger root juice along with the capsules, powder, and/or husks, when you start to take them. Drink a couple of liters (1 ounce of water for every 2 pounds of your body weight) of mineral-rich water, coconut water, fresh ginger root juice, and/ or more fresh, organic, vegetable juices throughout the day.

2. Starting on the second, third, or fourth day, depending on how long you are able to go with only liquids, start the combination of mixing 1 heaping teaspoon of green plant powder or capsules or a 6- to 8-ounce glass of freshly juiced organic greens with 1 teaspoon chia seeds and 1 heaping teaspoon or capsules of the husks with 1 teaspoon of the ground, raw pumpkin seeds with purified water (about 4 ounces) and drink it very quickly with one kalenite pill, one probiotic, and one digestive enzyme.
3. Drink an 8-ounce glass of pure water containing 1/8 teaspoon of high-quality sea salt immediately following. Drink as much high-quality water throughout the day as you can (1 ounce of water for every 2 pounds of your body weight).
4. Do this first thing in the morning on an empty stomach every day for three to 14 days minimum.
5. Do this at breakfast, lunch, and dinner (before 6 p.m.) every day for three to 14 days. If you are really serious about this, you can do it for 21 days.

Notes:

1. If you are extremely regular with bowel movements and feel like you have a very "clean" system, then you can have a separate cleanse mixture of psyllium husks. As an optional ingredient, you can add bentonite clay on its own along with this cleanse. The amount would be 1/8 teaspoon or less bentonite clay added

to the cleanse mixture. Lots of water or fluids need to be consumed when using these additional cleansing ingredients.

This mixture of psyllium husks and/or bentonite clay can remove more toxins, but should not be done if you have any kind of blockage or trouble moving the fiber through your body at all.

When using bentonite clay, don't take the green capsules; only take the psyllium husks and water. When using bentonite with psyllium, the bentonite "will absorb anything of nutritional value such as herbs, friendly bacteria, and vitamins, as well as toxins, bad bacteria and parasites. Be sure to wait 1 hour after doing a bentonite shake before taking anything nutritional."[34]

2. Psyllium husks expand very quickly when put into water and will turn into a thick glump you cannot drink. So, when you take it, either take it in capsule form or drink it really quickly once you add the water to it. This is what it will do in your stomach and is why you are taking it. It is great fiber and will make you feel full, as well as working like a large sponge to clean out your body's organs that it goes through. By absorbing toxins, it can really pull the toxins, as well as waste, from your body. You will go to the bathroom a few hours after you do this. If you feel bad, then you were very toxic, and you need to drink a lot of water to help flush out all of the toxins and help the fiber to continue on its journey out of your body.

You really should be going to the bathroom at least once for every time you eat. All food eaten should be efficiently digested, nutrients absorbed, and waste eliminated. If you are eating three times a day, then you should be having bowel movements three times a day. The more fiber you ingest, the easier and more efficiently the waste will be eliminated. There is not a set time period for this, but ideally it should be anywhere from three to 12 hours after each meal. You can test this by eating a meal of raw or slightly steamed red beets. The deep red color in the bowel movement will allow you to see when that meal is eliminated. This is an easy way to see if your body is eliminating quickly and efficiently. If you are not having regular bowel movements, then don't do the psyllium husks until you are. If you already started the cleanse and are not having regular bowel movements, then stop the fiber immediately and take only the greens until you are going regularly. If you feel uncomfortable and are not having bowel movements, you may want to get a colonics series to help get the system cleaned out and moving.

Drink lots of water; fresh, green, organic vegetable juices; and other liquids to keep the toxins, acid, and waste moving out of the body. This is so important! This cleanse is cleaning out of the inside of your body. With the removal of the plaque, waste, and debris, you will also be alkalizing your body and helping your body to maintain a healthier pH balance. Greens are highly alkalizing. This may seem like a lot of work or effort, but each time you do it, it will get easier, and you will start to feel better and have more energy! In situations where you feel you must have some food or really need something to chew, snacks or meals that consist of raw or lightly steamed, organic vegetables can be eaten about an hour before or after consuming the cleanse. You may also chew on some celery sticks or cucumber slices. Pure, whole sea salt and/or chia seeds may be sprinkled on the food. If you feel you must use some fat, then try using a little bit of coconut oil. The coconut oil can give you additional nourishment as well as ready energy.

For your convenience here is a list of some alkaline-forming foods, from most alkalizing to least alkalizing. There will be some variation in the order, depending on the food, its quality, and its source.

Mineral water and baking soda are highly alkalizing. Stevia is one of the most alkalizing sweeteners.

MOST:

Lemons
Watermelons
Cantaloupe
Limes
Parsley
Watercress
Sea kelp
Agar agar
Fresh vegetable juices
Asparagus
Dried dates, figs, and raisins
Mango
Melons
Pineapple
Endive
Kiwi fruit
Grapes
Passion fruit
Pears
Umeboshi plums

MODERATE:

- Kale
- Alfalfa sprouts
- Avocados
- Banana
- Berries
- Carrots
- Celery
- Garlic
- Gooseberries
- Grapefruit
- Guava
- Leafy green herbs and lettuce
- Nectarines
- Peaches
- Persimmons
- Sea salt
- Spinach
- Apples
- Apricots
- Fresh green beans
- Cabbage
- Broccoli
- Cauliflower
- Daikon radish
- Ginger
- Oranges
- Parsnip
- Pumpkins
- Raspberries
- Strawberries
- Squash
- Turnips
- Sweet corn
- Vinegar
- Almonds
- Artichokes
- Brussels sprouts
- Cherries
- Sprouts
- Cucumbers
- Honey
- Leeks
- Mushrooms
- Tomatoes
- Radish
- Raw goat's milk and whey
- Rhubarb
- Sesame seeds

Things that can help your body create an alkalizing environment are:

- Meditation
- Prayer
- Peace

Things that can cause the body to be in an acidic state are:

- Fear
- Worry
- Stress

Foods that are acidic in nature are:

- Sugars
- Meats
- Processed and refined foods
- Soft drinks
- Tobacco
- Alcohol

Grains, nuts, and beans are slightly acidic in nature.

Bentonite Clay

I add some bentonite clay to my cleanse on various occasions. Bentonite is a volcanic ash. It contains many minerals. It has a strong, negative polarized surface and edges, with a positive polarized surface that is a powerful electromagnetic field when hydrated, and it can attract and hold on to forms of radiation. It has the ability to pick up a great deal more than its own weight in positively charged particles. Dr. Jensen, ND, DC, PhD, suggested using bentonite to absorb radiation from bones. Bones are subjected to radiation through the use of X-rays, computers, television, and even radiation treatments for cancer. Bentonite clay has been used historically by American Indians for detoxifying and cleansing their bowels. Native Americans call it "Ee-Wah-Kee," meaning "the mud that heals." Bentonite is highly absorbable clay that has the ability to bind with toxins, drugs, and heavy metals, and draw them out of the body. You may wonder: If it is binding with these, does it bind with nutrients and pull them out, too? Some studies have demonstrated that, for bentonite clay to be harmful, a person would have to have 50% of his or her food intake be bentonite clay.[35]

Because of this, don't do this cleanse very often, and make sure that after the cleanse you add some extra nutrients to the body.

Some people put the liquid form of bentonite clay into their bath water (about a cup to a bathtub of water) to help pull out toxins from the body. The clay can be drying to the skin, though. The most effective type of bentonite clay is in a liquid colloidal state.

I had a cyst on my wrist and I didn't want to have surgery to remove it. I started researching natural ways to have it heal and I found bentonite clay. I started using it on a daily basis with my high-fiber cleanse, and within three weeks the cyst had disappeared.

The medical community has found clay to have amazing healing properties. One study by Arizona State University found:

> Unlike conventional antibiotics routinely administered by injection or pills, the so-called "healing clays" could be applied as rub-on creams or ointments to keep MRSA infections from spreading, according to a research duo from ASU's Biodesign Institute and College of Liberal Arts and Sciences.

> The clays also show promise against a wide range of other harmful bacteria, including those that cause skin infections and food poisoning, they add. Their study, one of the first to explore the antimicrobial activity of natural clays in detail, was presented at the 235th national meeting of the American Chemical Society, the world's largest scientific society....
>
> Clays have been used for thousands of years as a remedy for infected wounds, indigestion, and other health problems, either by applying clay to the skin or eating it. Cleopatra's famed beauty has been credited to her use of clay facials. Today, clays are still commonly used at health spas in the form of facials and mud baths. However, armed with new investigative tools, researchers Shelley Haydel and Lynda Williams are putting the clays to the test, scientifically.
>
> "Clays are little chemical drug-stores in a packet," says study co-leader Williams, a geochemist in the School of Earth and Space Exploration.[36]

"There are specific people who should refrain from the use of this substance. Women who are pregnant and senior citizens shouldn't consume bentonite clay or products that contain the material. You should also avoid taking bentonite clay within two hours of consumption of any medicine, including supplements."[37]

> Research at the Arizona State University, School of Life Sciences, report that a study of 20 clays from around the world, of types that included calcium bentonite, documents antimicrobial qualities in at least three samples, two of which are mined in the United States. The susceptible bacteria include methicillin resistant staphylococcus aureus, MRSA, a bacteria called Mycobacterium ulcerans, a tuberculosis-related organism that causes a flesh-digesting disease called Buruli. The bentonite

> clays also showed effectiveness against Escherecia coli and Salmonella, both of which are causes of foodborne illness. However, some clays, including calcium bentonite, are contaminated by ground water pollution and may also contain toxic mineral elements like arsenic. Do not use them for medical purposes unless you consult your doctor and use only materials known to be pure and clean.[38]

In conclusion, clay can have a very beneficial cleansing effect. Whether it is ingested or used on the skin, it is something to consider when doing a cleanse. (There is information about ordering in the Resources.)

Parasites

Bentonite clay and pumpkin seeds are ways to rid your body of parasites. We get parasites from many things, like ingesting dirt not completely washed off of food, eating meat, traveling in other countries, drinking water, and swimming in lakes or ponds.

Dr. Bernard Jensen, an expert in colon research and therapy, and other naturopaths, has recommended calcium bentonite clay for years as a vermifuge (parasite cleanser). He states that "the average person over 40 years of age has between 5 and 25 pounds of build-up in their colon.... Parasites of all sizes thrive in this undisposed residue of fecal matter, slowly but surely toxifying the whole body."[39]

If you have been traveling, swimming, or eating meat, it is very possible that you have picked up one or more somewhere. Dr. Peter Wina, chief of patho-biology at the Walter Reed Army Institute of Research says, "We have a tremendous parasitic problem right here in the U.S., it is just not being addressed."[40]

Joseph Sterling wrote in his newsletter, *Secrets of Robust Health*, that parasitic infection is common:

> Humans can play host to over 100 different kinds of parasites, ranging from microscopic to several feet long tapeworms. Contrary to popular belief, parasites are not restricted to our colon alone, but can be found in other parts of the body; the lungs,

> the liver, in the muscles and joints, in the esophagus, the brain, the blood, the skin and even in the eyes.[41]

Some common symptoms of parasitic infection are constipation, gas and bloating, diarrhea, back pain, joint and muscle pain, irritable bowel syndrome, allergies, insatiable hunger, itchy ears, nose, or anus, unpleasant sensations in the stomach, nervousness, grumpiness, chronic fatigue, lethargy or apathy, various skin problems, problems sleeping, nutritional deficiencies or anemia, problems with the immune system, teeth grinding or clenching, weight gain, forgetfulness, and blurry vision.

Those are all worth trying to fix, by doing a simple detoxification cleanse. In addition to simply adding bentonite clay and/or ground pumpkin seeds to the psyllium husk fiber cleanse, there are several anti-parasite cleanses on the market. The brands of Dr. Natura have a capsule called Paranil that you take on an empty stomach in different amounts for 30 days, first thing in the morning. This allows for the parasite to be expelled in all of the different stages of life, while living in the body. You really need to do the parasite cleanse for an entire three months (90 days), if doing this for the first time, because you want to make sure you rid the body of the parasite as it goes through all of the stages of life and isn't going to pop out in the future because it was in a stage that was not being addressed by the cleanse.

Here are a few of the products and brands available:

1. Perfect Food - Raw Greens by Garden of Life
2. Raw Kombucha by Garden of Life
3. Primadophilus Optima by Nature's Way
4. Green Magna by Green Foods
5. Whole Psyllium Husks by Yerba Prima
6. Kalenite Cleansing Herbs by Yerba Prima
7. Essential Enzymes by Source Natura
8. Paranil by Dr. Natura

Cilantro Cleanse for Metal Toxins

We all have some kinds of toxins in our bodies; metal toxins are harder to rid our bodies of. These are my instructions for doing a cilantro cleanse that can help detox the body.

Cilantro is a great detoxer of metal toxins. We get metal toxins in our bodies from a variety of places (for instance, dental fillings, aluminum deodorant, the aluminum foil we use in food preparation and storage, vaccinations, cadmium from secondhand smoke, polluted air, etc.). This is a bit of a challenge to do at first, but once you start doing it, it will get easier. I know, because I have done it. If you do this cleanse and you feel bad afterward, that is because it is pulling toxic metals from your cells and flushing them out into your blood stream. You really need to drink lots and lots of water to flush these toxins out. You may need to do this cleanse once a month until you can do it without feeling crummy at all. Then you know you have gotten the metal toxins out of your body really well.

Ingredients:

fresh organic cilantro

½ tsp. organic, extra-virgin olive oil

Directions:

1. Wash cilantro.
2. Put cilantro in a food processor and puree.
3. Mix pureed cilantro with olive oil.

Notes:

1. The oil helps it taste a little better and makes it easier to eat.
2. Store this in a glass container in the refrigerator. When storing, make certain you have a thin layer of olive oil over the top of the mixture. This "seals" the top to keep it fresh for a couple days.

Every morning for a week, eat at least 2 to 3 heaping teaspoons of the cilantro mixture. Do this first thing in the morning on an empty stomach. Chew it thoroughly and take a digestive enzyme with it for a more thorough cleanse. Wait at least 20 minutes before drinking water or eating anything else. For breakfast, the ideal choice would be to drink a glass of freshly juiced, organic green barley grass or wheatgrass, sprouts, ginger, and fresh vegetables. Drink a lot of water with a tiny bit of whole sea salt added to it, all day long. This is to help flush out the toxins that you have flushed out of the cells.

The key to any cleanse is to get the toxins you are pulling from the cells, completely out of the body, and not floating around in the blood stream.

Colonic Cleanse

A colonic is a type of cleanse that many people recommend for someone with a high degree of inflammation, constipation, and/or plaque in his or her intestines. It is a rinse of the intestine with water. Water is used to cleanse the layers of the walls of the intestine. Each time it is done, another layer of plaque or waste can be washed out of the lining of the colon and the intestines. If the body is not eliminating meals efficiently after each meal, there may be some blockage in the intestinal tract. Some people find it so useful they continue to do it once a month or more just to stay clean.

Natalia Rose, one of my teachers in cleansing, and master colon therapist Gil Jacobs believe in this method. If you have been a consumer of processed foods, fried foods, or trans fats, or if you are/were a meat eater, then your body may have some blockages, or plaque or debris lodged in the intestinal tract or colon.

Having a colonic is actually very easy. The gravity method colonic is the type of equipment that Gil and Natalia recommend. People say, "I got a colonoscopy and it was fine." A colonoscopy doesn't really clean out the lining of the intestines. It is like a bullet going through a gun. It doesn't pull out the toxins or plaque embedded in the lining of the intestines. Colonics actually wash out the debris, plaque, and whatever else is stuck in the layers of the intestinal wall. When receiving a colonic, a client reclines in a large chair, and water is slowly introduced into the colon by a narrow tube. The warm water washes up very slowly, and there is only a small quantity. Then the water runs out of the colon, being released to flow out though a tube and go directly into the septic system. The hydrotherapist answers questions, guides, or assists whenever needed.

When I took Natalia Rose's cleansing class in New York, Gil Jacobs explained that a laxative will do nothing for the normal person who is eating fairly well except release the very newest waste, and then drive the older waste deeper into the tissue and make it harder to remove. The laxative will irritate the bowels.

Enemas are another way to remove waste from the bowels. These can work well and get waste to come out of the tissue. Enemas are recommended by Natalia Rose. She says that if you wake up in the morning, have a bowel movement, and pull in your gut, and it is almost to your spine, then you have an empty and clean intestine. If you cannot do this, then your intestines are full of undigested waste stuck in the tissues like cement. After years and years of eating meals that are not completely digested or moved out of the body, there are layers and layers of waste built up. Gil Jacobs and Natalia Rose say a person who grew up eating a "standard American diet" of bread, meat, trans fats, sugar, and junk food could get a colonic every week for the rest of his or her life and still not have all of the waste completely removed from the colon.

A raw food diet will help awaken the body and the waste, and help get it to move out. Changing the diet to be one of a mostly raw food will help, because the food is more likely to be completely or close to completely digested, and the body will start to cleanse itself of toxins because of the anti-oxidant-rich food and fiber. When the colon and intestinal tract are cleaned up and running free and clear, the whole body will start to work in harmony. Many people will find their joint problems, headaches, back aches, skin problems, hair problems, and so forth simply disappear when they finally get their colon and intestines clean and oxygenated.

Natalia Rose recommends the following colon therapists:

Chakra 17 West
Portland, Oregon
(503) 493–9656
www.chakra17.com

Chakra 17 East
401 East Thirty-Fourth St.
New York, NY
(212) 679–6576
www.chakra17.com

Gil Jacobs
528 Fifth St.
New York, NY
(212) 254–5279

Prana Brooklyn
Contact: Donna Perrone
825 Caton Ave.
Brooklyn, NY
(646) 435–7277

Digestion

Good digestion is extremely important for optimum health. When we eat, we actually begin the digestion process when we start to chew our food. Because digestion actually starts in our mouth, it is very important to chew our food well. Chewing will get your digestive juices going.

Chew something, even just one bite, before drinking a drink, like a smoothie (which many people these days tend to have as a meal), so you can get the digestive juices flowing in the mouth.

Eating a piece of fruit or a few raw vegetables 10 or 15 minutes before a meal will help you feel fuller faster, because it takes your mind about 15 minutes to know you are full. So, if you eat something about 10 or 15 minutes before eating a meal, your mind and stomach will already start becoming in sync with your digestive progress; there won't be a gap of time before being full and actually having your brain know you are full. My advice for optimum digestion is to eat slowly and to not eat while standing up, walking, or driving. Sit down, savor the flavor, and try to have a peaceful atmosphere when you are eating so your body can concentrate on digestion efficiently. Also, don't drink beverages with a meal. They water down the digestive juices so they aren't as acidic and can make it harder for your body to digest the food you are eating. As we age, we have fewer digestive enzymes. This means our body cannot digest food as well. There are some digestive enzymes you can take before a meal to help your body digest food more completely.

Thoroughly digesting food is critically important for maintaining a healthy body. Dr. Alan Chen, my acupuncturist/chiropractor in Plano, Texas, is a 14th-generation Chinese doctor. He told me that he takes three digestive enzymes before every meal. The better we digest our food, the more readily the body will be able to absorb the nutrients, and the less waste will be sitting in the intestines creating problems. In my opinion, high-quality digestive enzymes can be very beneficial for anyone who would like to aid his or her body in the digestion process.

Dining Away from Home

At a restaurant, if you care that the food you eat is vegetarian, you need to ask questions. One day my son said, "Mom, don't ask or there won't be anything for you to eat." Sometimes that is actually right. I have been to many Mexican food restaurants that put lard (animal fat) and beef or chicken broth in absolutely everything they serve. They cook the chips and tortillas in lard, bake the beans with pork or with lard, and cook the rice and cheese dip with animal broth and/or lard. They even put meat juice in the pico de gallo and salsa. That leaves me with a choice of lettuce and a sliced avocado, or something like that. If you really want to know, then ask.

I always ask if the vegetables are cooked with meat. I have ordered green beans, only to find out they were cooked with bacon. I have ordered salads that have had bacon on them or in the salad dressing. I always ask, and I tell my server that I do not want any meat, chicken, or fish of any kind in any of my food. I always say specifically "beef, chicken, or fish," because many people think that chicken and fish are parts of a vegetarian diet. Be specific about what you do not want. You may also request food that is free of MSG and sulfites. I ask what oil they cook the food in, what the soup base is, and what the salad dressing has in it. I would rather know what I am eating than be surprised later. It's amazing how hard it is to get whole, real food today at restaurants, though more and more today can accommodate you with healthier food. You can simply say that you are on a special diet for your health. This often makes people more accommodating. There are so many health issues today that require a special diet (a lot of them probably because of all of these additives!), so it won't seem like such an unusual request. Most restaurants can at least serve you a plate of steamed vegetables.

I have found that many times I can order the side dishes on a menu. They are fairly large portions (and are usually less expensive). For our family, we order a few of those and split them. Even barbecue and steak restaurants usually have really terrific side dishes, which makes dining there with others really easy.

Many times, I will take a small bottle of my own salad dressing, just in case the place has unhealthy salad dressing choices. I may also eat a little bit before I go, just to be sure I am not starving when we arrive.

I have also taken small baggies with a few carrots or crackers, just to guarantee that I won't starve if there are no healthy choices on the menu. Most restaurants today still have no whole-grain crackers or bread, and many of the salad dressings are full of chemicals and sugar. When you go to a large party or formal affair, it is easy to tell the wait staff that you are a vegetarian and ask them to bring a vegetable plate. They usually are prepared for this, and it is really no problem most of the time.

When I go to someone's home for a dinner party, I take a dish of food as my hostess gift. This way I know there will be something I can eat, and maybe some of the other guests will enjoy it as well. For a cookout I usually take a pack of vegetarian burgers or hot dogs and some whole-grain buns. Make sure you get to eat some of the food that you brought before everyone eats it all; that has happened to me many times!

At parties and/or places where I am not sure there will be any food, I take some food with me, like a raw food bar, a bag of raisins, or trail mix. If I am going to a late-night party and I am not sure there will be food, I often take a serving of my high-fiber detox cleanse before I go. The psyllium husks expand and fill me, and I am not as hungry throughout the event.

Many people do not consider fish or chicken "meat." You may have to make sure people understand this. I said yes to pizza one day at a restaurant. When it arrived, it was covered with shrimp. They thought that a vegetarian "doesn't eat cows." They didn't even consider chicken or fish as foods I don't eat. There are many people who say they are vegetarian and eat fish and chicken. By definition, people who eat fish and chicken are not vegetarian. I will simply say I am a full practicing vegetarian, and I don't eat creatures with parents.

Enzymes, Energy, and Detoxification

Live enzymes regenerate our cells and feed our bodies. In the publication, "The Status of Food Enzymes in Digestive and Metabolism," Dr. Edward Howell wrote:

> It is no longer warranted to consider vitality and life energy as intangible forces. The available evidence does not justify a placid continuance of nihilistic attitude toward the vital forces operating in the living organism. Enzymes emerge as the true yardstick of vitality. Enzymes offer an important means of calculating the vital energy of an organism. That which has been referred to as vitality, vital force... probably is synonymous with that which has been known as enzyme activity....[42]

"Dr. Howell was not alone in holding this concept, which is equally shared by prominent scholars like Professor Moore of the University of Oxford in England, professor Willstatter of Munich in Germany and Northrop of Rockefellar Institute for Medical Research."[43] As Dr. Howell explained, and what many people believe and are practicing today would say: It is all about enzymes! The more organic, living, whole foods we eat, the more ammunition and fuel our bodies have to nourish, heal, and purge themselves of toxins that we can accumulate throughout the day. Live (raw) food that hasn't been heated or processed over 105 degrees is living food. Heating and processing food destroys the live enzymes in it.

We have a limited supply of digestive enzymes in our system, and making new ones as we age becomes more and more difficult and/or impossible. When we are young, we have a natural abundance of enzymes. By the time we are elderly, we have lost over half of our enzymes. Different foods like meats, not properly chewing our food, pathogenic microbes, and chewing gum all make our body utilize more of our digestive enzymes and deplete the amount we have to use. According to Dr. Edward Howell, our digestive system is only able to digest about half of the food we eat.[44] An apple that has not been irradiated (which destroys the enzymes) will have a ratio of about 40 to 60 enzymes. This means that the apple will provide the live enzymes for breaking down for digestion about 40 to 60 percent of that apple, before our body has to produce the enzymes or acid to complete the digestion process.

Cooked food, on the other hand, has no living enzymes in it to help the body digest it. Therefore the body is forced to use its precious supply of digestive enzymes in order to break down the food, in order to utilize any of the nutrients. This causes stress on the digestive system, the pancreas, and the immune system. When cooked, or "dead," foods are eaten, the body has to break down 100 percent of that food, creating a depletion of digestive enzymes. In his book *Enzyme Nutrition,* Dr. Howell said, "We know that decreased enzyme levels are found in a number of chronic ailments, such as allergies, skin disease and even serious diseases like diabetes and other severe diseases."[45]

Let me expand on this. First, food is chewed in the mouth. Saliva starts the digestion process. The better food is chewed, the better the food is able to begin the process of being broken down. Then, food is swallowed and goes into the upper stomach, where it should stay to predigest about an hour. Foods that are really pure and clean, like fresh, organic fruit, will be digested the fastest. There are no live enzymes supplied by the body for this stage of digestion. Then food passes into the lower part of the stomach, where the body provides hydrochloric, trypsin, and pepsin acid to break down food before it moves into the small intestinal tract, where digestive enzymes from the pancreas are supposed to complete the digestion process. When food is digested, the nutrients are absorbed through the intestinal wall into the blood steam.

One of the main problems with health today is the lack of complete digestion of food. If the food we eat isn't broken down properly, it won't be able to be absorbed properly or completely by our body. We absorb most of our nutrients in the intestinal tract through the intestinal wall, when food is not properly broken down in the stomach, it goes into the intestines too large to be completely digested and then absorbed. Because of this, the undigested food sits there and begins to rot. When this occurs, the body tries to protect itself from the rotting food and the putrid acid it creates by building up a plaque wall inside the walls of the intestine, so that it won't make holes in the intestinal wall and have the dying bacteria get through into the body. (Sometimes it does get through, resulting in inflammation and disease.) This plaque, built up over years, can be so thick that if healthy food does get into the intestine in a proper condition, it can't be absorbed because the plaque prevents the nutrients from getting through.

Dr. Howell researched diets of cooked versus raw food. In his studies of rats, he found that rats on a raw, living food diet lived about 50 percent longer than rats on cooked food. His studies with people in a sanitarium led him to conclude: "It is impossible to get people fat on raw foods...regardless of the calorie intake."[46] Along with that conclusion, Dr. Anthony Cheung, FRCP, noted:

> Dr. Howell's use of Food Enzymes suggests that the supply of human enzymes is limited at birth. The faster we consume our enzymes, the shorter will be our life span. Raw food is a good source of food enzymes. Ingestion of raw food or enzyme supplements will lessen the work of our digestive system so that more energy is reserved for other metabolic activities.[47]

The Pottinger Cat Study, an extensive, 10-year study with about 900 cats conducted by Dr. Francis Pottinger, studied the effects of raw food versus cooked food on the health and well-being of the test subjects. He had two groups of cats. One group was fed a diet of raw meat and milk (which had live enzymes and probiotics as a natural part of the food), and the other group was given cooked meat and pasteurized milk (where the food's enzymes and probiotic nature had been killed with heat). He wanted to show the difference over time of a diet of cooked, processed food versus raw foods. What he found was that the cats that were eating raw food remained healthy and disease-free for generation after generation. The cats on the cooked-food diet slowly started to get lazy and have degenerative diseases. The second generation of these cooked-food-fed cats got mid-life degenerative diseases, and the third generation had very serious diseases like blindness, shorter life spans, and the incapability to produce offspring.

Eat whole, organic, raw, living food. These foods will provide nutrient-dense, live enzymes that really feed your body. Isn't this why we eat food, anyway? Nourishing our bodies should be a major reason we are eating food in the first place. What we consume is what becomes our blood, cells, skin, hair, and so on. Our well-being depends on the quality of our food. Food starts to die the moment it is picked. Food we buy at the supermarket is probably at least five days old. The fresher the food, the more alive it is. The enzymes will be more vibrant and rich in nutrients. Locally grown or home-grown, fresh, organic fruits, vegetables, nuts, seeds, and grains will give the body more nutrient-dense, enzyme-rich food to process, absorb, and turn into the body cells. It is all about energy. Fresh food is more vibrant. Therefore we are more vibrant when we eat it. We are, after all, what we eat.

These foods are also more alkalizing. Processed foods are very acidic. Freshly juiced grasses, fruits, and vegetables are full of anti-oxidants and nutrients, and are highly alkalizing and oxygenating. Drinking these can help flush the toxins out of the body, feed the body on a deep cellular level with live enzymes, and alkalize the body. Drink fresh juice within 20 minutes of juicing in order to get the maximum nutrient benefits. Our bodies need to maintain a pH balance of around 7.2. If we eat too many acidic foods, our bodies do all kinds of things in order to adjust, one of which is to pull calcium out of the bones. A diet high in fresh fruits and vegetables (juiced or in whole-food form) contributes to a more alkaline-rich diet, which can help with the maintenance of the pH in the body. Disease can thrive in an acidic environment, so maintaining the pH is important for health.

Take a good digestive enzyme supplement a few minutes before each meal and/or eat lots of fresh sprouts daily with every meal. This will aid in your body's ability to break down the food you are eating. Digestive enzymes are critical to our health.

> Digestive enzymes help the digestive process to assimilate proteins, carbohydrates and fat. In 1930, only 80 enzymes had been identified; in 1970, more than 1,300 enzymes were known. By now, over 4,000 have been found—and counting. If we do not get enzymes with our daily food to aid our digestion, our body's digestive enzymes will carry the complete load, depleting the limited resources.

> Enzymes have a vital activity factor that is exhaustible, and our capacity to make enzymes is limited. It appears that the safest answer is to sprout all your intake of seeds and grains. In this process the inhibitors are neutralized and life process commences with enzymes that are alive and active.[48]

Dr. William S. Peavy, who has an MA in horticulture from the University of California and a PhD from Kansas State University, used to write for the *El Paso Times*, and has over a hundred published articles and a few books, said:

> All of us have a limited capacity to produce enzymes. Like the engine of the car that has a limited capacity to produce horsepower. And this capacity declines with age. It is this capacity which we are born with, that determines our maximum potential life span. Some are born with a greater potential life span, and others less. In any case, as we age, in general, our body is able to produce less and less enzymes. It is this general decline in enzyme activity in our body that is a fundamental cause of aging. When enzyme activity gets too low, the process of death occurs.[49]

> Sprouts have large amounts of enzymes that can contribute to the amount of enzymes in the stomach that can contribute to the digestion process. Digestive enzyme supplements from whole food form can help as well. Dr. Chen, a 14th generation Chinese Doctor that I use, told me that he takes 3 digestive enzymes with every meal. He takes digestion and enzymes really seriously.[50]

Slow down and chew your food. Chew food very slowly, mindfully, and completely. It seems so silly to realize that this is a simple way to help our health. In our stressful, fast-paced life, we don't take time to actually chew or even truly enjoy eating our food. This fast-food mentality puts much stress on the body and the digestive system. It is no wonder that there are so many diseases that are associated with the digestive system. Chewing is an enjoyable process. We actually start digesting the food while it is in our mouth. The brain knows what enzymes to use in the stomach by what it detects being chewed in the mouth. This is a reason that gum is not a good idea: It tricks the mind into thinking that we are going to be digesting food soon. It calls out the enzymes, and the precious supply of digestive enzymes is wasted. We will use up our enzymes in this way. Live enzymes are a key to staying healthy and youthful. We want to do everything we can to protect the ones we have, and supplement them when we can by eating foods with live enzymes and/or taking additional live enzyme supplements.

Chewing slowly can be enjoyable and satisfying. It takes the brain about 10 to 15 minutes to become aware of the stomach being full. If we are not chewing our food properly or slowly, we can overeat. Take this seriously. Slow down and really chew food, which will help your body produce the enzymes needed to digest it much more thoroughly.

Exercise and the Lymphatic System

Exercise gets the body oxygenated and helps the lymphatic system keep moving as well as draining. The lymphatic system is part of the immune system. It is comprised of a network called lymphatic vessels. These vessels, similar to blood vessels, carry a clear fluid called lymph. These vessels carry the lymphatic fluids unidirectionally toward the heart. While the blood stream is pumped by the heart, it is circulated throughout the body and is cleansed by the kidneys. The lymphatic system doesn't have a pump to help it keep moving. The lymphatic system moves through the body in an upward system through the body and extremities and up toward the neck, where it enters the subclavian veins and becomes part of the plasma and blood stream once more. The lymph nodes along the way are where the lymph is filtered or cleansed. When any part of this system gets clogged, it can cause inflammation. Inflammation leads to disease.

I read the book *Dressed to Kill: The Link Between Breast Cancer and Bras* about 15 years ago. Written by medical anthropologist Sydney Singer and her assistant, Soma Grismaijer, it talked about the lymphatic system and how constrictive clothing (like bras and belts) and a lack of exercise could be causing various types of cancer and disease by creating sluggish or clogged lymph nodes. There is three times as much lymphatic fluid as blood, and it is a critical part of our immune system. Some signs of a compromised or clogged lymphatic system include swollen hands or feet, painful swelling of the lymph nodes, any type of arthritis or bronchitis, lack of energy or mental clarity, trouble sleeping, cysts or fibrous tumors, an inability to recover quickly from viral infections, or, last but not least, cancer.

Exercise so that the body's lymphatic system is able to stay clog-free. The movements of muscles stimulate the flow of the lymphatic system. Lymphatic massages are helpful, especially if you feel you have some clogged lymph nodes, but exercise that keeps the body moving and the lymphatic system draining is the easiest way to keep this system healthy and clog-free on a regular basis. Try to do something you enjoy. Don't let exercise be a chore or work. Make it fun and let it lift your spirits.

Stress is known as a "silent killer." Exercise is shown to help relieve stress. Walking, biking, bouncing on a trampoline or rebounder, yoga, dance, roller blading—whatever you prefer, make exercise a priority in life and make your life healthier, less stressful, and more fun.

Fats: What's the Skinny?

When people tell me they need protein, I think they really need good fat in their diet. Their bodies are craving "good" fat. Fat in our food can make it taste more rich and satisfying. The advertising industry would have us believe that fat is bad or fattening, but really good fat can be critical to our health and our weight. Many low-fat or fat-free products are filled with salt, sugar, chemical additives, MSG, and so forth in order to make up for the lack of fat. Fat is a critical component to our health. Fat actually tells the body how to utilize protein and carbohydrates. Good fats are vital for good brain health. (When I refer to "good" fats I am talking about raw, unprocessed, organic fats in their natural form.) Trans fats should always be avoided completely. Trans fats are hydrogenated fats that have been chemically changed into a non-natural or abnormal condition. They will stay solid at room temperature and have an extremely long shelf life. These are unhealthy even in tiny amounts.

Essential fatty acids are called essential because they are not made by our body and must be obtained through the diet. Omega 3s and 6s are the specific essential fatty acids I'll address in this book. We should all try to have a balance of Omega 3 and Omega 6 fats in our diet every day. Many doctors recommend a ratio of 3 to 1 (with Omega 6 being the 3, and Omega 3 being the 1). However, a couple doctors at the Institute of Integrative Nutrition affiliated with Columbia University said the ratio really should be closer to 1 to 1. Most Americans get much more Omega 6s than 3s, so it may be important for you really work on getting the proper amount of Omega 3 essential fatty acids into your diet. Omega 3s help with the prevention of many health problems (because of their anti-inflammatory properties): heart disease, rheumatoid arthritis, macular degeneration, asthma, eczema, other immune dysfunctions, and cancer. Omega 3s also help with improving memory and can help improve mood. A deficiency may appear as inflammation, water retention, and high blood pressure.

I like raw, cold-pressed nut and seed oils. Pumpkin, walnut, flax, sesame, almond, hemp, and macadamia nut are some of my favorites. I only use them in recipes where they are not being heated, or, if I do add them, it is after they have been cooked and cooled down. The foods you make and eat will be more satisfying and delicious with an added health benefit. If you are worried about weight gain, these good fats can actually help with weight loss. The bad fats and other additives to the processed foods are what can cause ill health and weight problems.

Coconut oil is a type of "nut" fat. It is a saturated fat, a highly chemically stable fat, and resistant to peroxidation and rancidity. It is highly effective as an anti-oxidant. The Natural Gourmet Institute for Food and Health always used coconut oil whenever cooking with heat. I learned this when I was there taking my health-supportive cooking class. (Very few oils handle heat well. Certain coconut oils handle high heat very well. Read labels and make certain that you are purchasing the type that is meant to handle whichever cooking method you require. Some that are more refined will say whether they are meant for cooking with high heat.) Coconut oil is a unique, healthy fat, and I have found it to be a healthy and safe oil for any cooking recipe. Coconut oil is seen in most parts of the world as the super-food of fats. It is a unique saturated fat and a medium-chain fatty acid in that it doesn't need pancreatic enzymes or bile in order for the body to process it. This means that it is easily absorbed by the body. Coconut oil nourishes the body and the medium -chained fatty acids provide a good source of energy. Also, the lauric acid in coconut oil is a natural immune system booster.[51] For years many people thought coconut oil was bad for health because it raised cholesterol, but, in actuality, it provides "good" cholesterol (HDL). Pure coconut oil is known as a functional food and has many benefits besides its nutritional value, among them:

- Promoting your heart health
- Supporting your immune system health
- Supporting a healthy metabolism
- Providing you with an immediate energy source
- Helping to keep your skin healthy and youthful-looking
- Supporting the proper functioning of your thyroid gland[52]

Coconut oil appears to be unique in its ability to help with brain function. Recently I read about Dr. Mary T. Newport curing her husband of Alzheimer's disease. She began adding coconut oil to his diet and asserted this to be one of the main components of his cure. So, what is Alzheimer's disease and why would coconut oil help? Alzheimer's disease "appears to be a type of diabetes of the brain and it's a process that starts happening at least 10 or 20 years before you start having symptoms and it's very similar to type 1 or type 2 diabetes in that you develop a problem with insulin. In this case, insulin problems prevent brain cells from accepting glucose, their primary fuel. Without it, they eventually die. But there is an alternative fuel: ketones, which cells easily accept. Ketones metabolized in the liver after you eat medium-chain triglycerides, like those found in coconut oil."[53]

Throughout this book, I have coconut oil in many of my recipes. Make sure you purchase organic, extra-virgin, pure coconut oil. You do not want to purchase or confuse pure coconut oil with a hydrogenated or trans fat variety.

Canola is a brand name. It is a plant in Canada developed from the rapeseed plant, which is a member of the mustard family. It is used in many products and foods because it is apparently low in saturated fats and has a high proportion of monosaturated fats. I have seen advertisements that say it is all right to use when cooking with heat. Never heat oil (any oil) over its smoking point. The smoke produced can be toxic. Many foods that are prepared at restaurants, stores, and bakeries have canola oil as an ingredient.

The erucic acid levels in the rapeseed oil are said to be toxic. Rapeseed oil contains about 30 to 60 percent erucic acid. Canola oil has been developed to contain a range of erucic acid of 1.2 to .3 percent. Canola oil is fairly new and hasn't been around long enough to have its effects on humans and animals studied and understood completely. Canola oil has been subject to much controversy. It is up to you to decide if canola oil is right for you.

Olive oil is a wonderful, unique ingredient in that it is an Omega 9 oil, monosaturated fat, long-chained fatty acid, and the only vegetable oil that can be pressed and used in its pure form. The key ingredient found in olive oil is oleic acid. Some studies have shown it to aid in cancer protection.[51]

It is a good fat and a staple in the healthy Mediterranean diet. Olive oil can become rancid if heated or stored improperly. It needs to be kept cool (or refrigerated) and away from light. (In fact, all nut, seed, and vegetable oils should be kept refrigerated and away from light.) Olive oil should be used only with non-cooking recipes and food preparation, unless it says on the label that it is meant to handle high heat. More refined varieties of olive oils can handle certain high temperatures. When olive oil (or any oil, for that matter) is heated beyond what is known as the smoke point, the oil can actually become toxic. George Mateljan (biologist, businessman, and nutritionist who is best known for his book, *The World's Healthiest Foods*) told journalist Jen Weigel of *Chicago Now* "that olive oil should be heated below 250 degrees otherwise toxic fumes can be created from oil that is overheated. People are inhaling this smoke every day when they think it's being healthy, but in reality, the smoke from heated olive oil is full of toxins."[55] Ms. Weigel followed up with George about olive oil. She said:

> I emailed George to ask him about this, as well as whether or not you can bake with olive oil without the toxic smoke, since that was also a concern to many. He said that yes indeed, he does not recommend heating olive oil above 200–250 degrees Fahrenheit, **not** Centigrade. He says that you can bake with olive oil up to 350F degrees, and it will not smoke because the molecules are surrounded by moisture and dough.[56]

When Weigel had some people questioning her article, she went on to say:

> Dr. Oz did his food "Hall of Shame" episode, and suddenly, I was validated. He listed many foods to avoid in order to be your best self, and stay healthy. In this video clip from Oprah.com, he mentions that you should NOT cook healthy oils, because "when you have healthy oils, and you cook with them, you damage them…. Healthy oils would be olive oil, sesame oil, canola oil, or flaxseed oil."[57]

Choose organic, extra-virgin olive oil, which is from the first press of the olive, if you are using olive oil for non-cooking recipes. "While olive oil can and should be a healthy part of your diet, what most people do not appreciate is that olive oil should not be used to cook with."[58] Extra-virgin olive oil has more Vitamin E in it than other types of olive oil. Olive oil "is a monounsaturated fat and contains major health benefits because of its vitamin E and A, chlorophyll, magnesium, squalene and a host of other cardio-protective nutrients. It has also been shown to reduce some cancers, as well as rheumatoid arthritis."[59]

Hemp oil contains significant amounts of Omega 3s and Omega 6s. Hemp oil also contains significant amounts of Vitamin E, which is important for the thyroid gland. One easy thing you can do for your diet is to freshly grind hemp or flax seeds and add them to recipes for an extra benefit of omega oils as well as protein and fiber.

Flax seeds are one of the best sources of Omega 3 essential fatty acids. Flax seeds are rich with alpha-linolenic acid, fiber, and lignans. Lignans are phytoestrogens or plant compounds that have an estrogen-like effect with anti-oxidant properties. These lignans can help stabilize hormone levels and reduce PMS and menopause symptoms. They can also potentially help reduce the risk of developing prostate or breast cancer. The alpha-linolenic acid is anti-inflammatory. It promotes the lowering of the C-Reactive Protein in the blood, which is a biomarker of inflammation. Freshly grind flax seeds when using them to get the full benefit of the oil. Do not buy flax seeds that are already ground. Store flax seeds in a dry, waterproof container. Always store ground seeds in the refrigerator.

Chia seeds are an ancient seed cultivated for thousands of years in Mexico. The word means "strength." Aztec history says that the warriors could live off of one teaspoon of chia seeds for a whole day.[60] Unlike flax seeds and hemp seeds, chia seeds do not have to be ground up in order for the body to utilize the nutrients and oils, making them much easier for the body to use. Chia seeds have more Omega 3 fatty acids than Atlantic salmon, but unlike the salmon, chia seeds also are about 10% Omega 6 oil, so they are a more perfect balance of omega fats. Chia seeds are 3 Omega 3s to 1 Omega 6. Along with the rich omega oils, chia seeds also have four times more calcium than milk (1 ounce of chia has 179 mg. calcium and 1 ounce of whole milk has 36 mg. calcium), more anti-oxidants than fresh blueberries, and more protein, calcium, and fiber than flax seeds. Chia seeds are one of the best nutrient-dense super-foods around.

NOTE: Chia seeds, ground flax seeds, or ground hemp seeds can provide Omega 3s. You can also buy Omega 3 flax seed oil at the grocery store. Omega 6 essential fatty acids need to be balanced with Omega 3 essential fatty acids. An excess of Omega 6 can cause water retention, raised blood pressure, and increased blood clotting.

Almonds are extremely high in Omega 6 (1,800 Omega 6 oils to 1 Omega 3 oil), so make sure to balance that with a high source of Omega 3. Good sources of Omega 6 are safflower oil, sunflower oil, sesame seed oil, hemp oil, pumpkin oil, walnut oil, almond oil, wheat germ oil, and evening primrose oil.

Clarified butter (ghee) is butter that has had the milk solids removed. It has been used for centuries in ancient Ayurvedic medicine. It is supposed to enhance the essence that governs the tissues of the body and balance hormones. Ayurvedic medicine traditions say that ghee provides assistance in healing injuries and gastro-intestinal problems, and in being disease-resistant. Dr. Rudolph Ballentine, MD, did some studies and found that it contained butyric acid, has properties that are anti-viral and anti-cancer, and can also help in the prevention of Alzheimer's disease. This clarified butter is usually sold in the Asian/Indian food area or in the baking goods area of stores. I love the buttery flavor of ghee and use it at the end of many recipes, in small amounts, just to add that touch of butter flavor to the coconut oil or other fat I used.

Choose organic, whole-food, cold-pressed, non-processed vegetarian "good" fats and enjoy your food. Don't feel guilty about adding the healthy fat to recipes. Your body and your brain will be glad you did!

"Think of the fierce energy concentrated in an acorn! You bury it in the ground, and it explodes into an oak! Bury a sheep, and nothing happens but decay."

~ George Bernard Shaw

Fermented Foods

Fermented foods date back in the Middle East as far as 1000 BC. Cleopatra was known to eat pickles made with vinegar and thought they made her more beautiful. Asian and Western cultures ferment foods. In Asia, it is miso, kimchi, umeboshi, kombucha, and soy sauce. In the Western culture, it is cheese, pickles, yogurt, relishes, and sauerkraut. Fermented foods are more easily digestible, and they contain nutrients such as folic acid, riboflavin, biotin, thiamin, and niacin. Fermented foods increase the levels of usable amino acids, which help with calcium absorption and muscle-building protein. They have anti-oxidant properties and contribute to positive flora growth in the intestinal tract, which boosts the immune system. Fermentation is usually done by using vinegar and water, salt and water, or air with a food or beverage. The vinegar or salt is mixed with the food or beverage, then left to sit and rest. Bacteria will then begin to work with the combination and it will ferment, creating beneficial bacteria that we then ingest with the food or beverage. These beneficial bacteria support our immune system and help keep non-beneficial bacteria in control. If no beneficial bacteria are present, then non-beneficial bacteria can take over. Anyone who has taken antibiotics should replenish the good bacteria in their system. antibiotics can wipe out all of the good bacteria in a person's system. So, consuming fermented foods rich with their beneficial bacteria can make a huge difference in rebuilding a strong immune system.

I try to have, at the very least, one tablespoon of a fermented food or liquid every day in some food that I eat or even by itself. (Many times, I will have a good deal more than just that tablespoon.) This is such a small amount, but at the very least I put some fermented foods or drinks on a daily basis into my system and help replenish the beneficial bacteria in my body.

Candida Albicans

Many people today are walking around with this yeast growing in their bodies and they don't even know it. They may feel "not so great" and don't know why, and they look fine. Yeast is a bit insidious and feeds on sugar. *Candida Albicans* is yeast-like fungal organism found in tiny amounts in the normal human intestinal tract. A healthy beneficial flora (bacteria) that is part of the immune system usually keeps it in balance.

A weakened immune system is a major cause of the over-growth of this yeast-like fungal problem. The immune system is compromised by the excessive use of antibiotics, steroids (like Prednisone), and oral contraceptives, high acidic pH levels in our body from poor diet and stress, hormone imbalances, and exposure to environmental toxins (often molds). Over-exposure to any of these things can cause fungal yeast overgrowth. This can be extremely serious. According to a Harvard study, it is more common than we might think and with serious side effects. From the *Harvard Gazette*:

> Known scientifically as *Candida albicans*, "it is, by far, the most predominant fungus involved in human disease," according to Julia Koehler, a Harvard fellow in infectious diseases, "Fungal infections acquired in U.S. hospitals doubled from 1980 to 1990, and *Candida* was responsible for almost 60 percent of them. It killed one of every three people with a bloodstream infection."[61]

There are two levels of *Candida* overgrowth: *Mucocutaneous Candidiasis,* which infects the mucous membranes, and *Disseminated Candidiasis,* which involves the blood stream and can infect the organs of the body. This second type can be dangerous and life-threatening. Early treatment in both types may help avoid further complications.

When the immune system is weak and the beneficial bacteria (like acidophilus) that support the immune system are wiped out from the use of various things like antibiotics, the immune system does not have the capabilities to keep the bad bacteria and normal levels of yeast in check. When this occurs, the normal yeast present in our bodies, called *Candida,* can change from being beneficial yeast into being harmful fungus. This fungal yeast can quickly grow out of the balance in our body and overwhelm the beneficial flora (bacteria) that normally keep natural yeast levels in a healthy balance.

This new fungal form of yeast develops rhizoids (long, burrowing legs). These rhizoids can puncture the colon and the walls of the small intestine. These rhizoids create a chemical waste that can spread throughout the body, causing serious, chronic conditions. Leaky Gut Syndrome is one of the results, along with partially digested proteins getting into the blood stream and being transported throughout the body. This combination of protein and yeast becomes toxic. Once this yeast infection has access to the whole body, the result is *Systemic Candida.*

Some symptoms of *Systemic Candida* are increasing allergies to foods (gluten or celiac problems can be a direct result of *Candida* overgrowth), vaginal yeast infections (also known as vaginal thrush), constant fatigue, brain fog (when you can't think straight), oral thrush (a white film on the tongue, especially first thing in the morning), bad breath or a bad taste in the mouth, abdominal pain (intestinal *Candida*), bloating and indigestion, constant carbohydrate and/or sweets cravings, joint pain or arthritis types of pain, chronic sinus drainage (which medicines like antibiotics aren't able to help), weight gain (or loss) and the inability to change it, fungus on the fingernails or toenails, and personal area infections.

You are dealing with *Candida* yeast overgrowth if you experiencing even one or two of these conditions.

According to Dr. Mark Hyman:

> Medical students learn about fungal and yeast problems, but only in a limited way. They know that AIDS patients have severe yeast and fungal infections and need long-term anti-fungal treatment. People with diabetes tend to grow yeast because yeast likes sugar. Babies get thrush and need anti-fungal treatment. Women get vaginal Candida yeast infections. All of these are well-accepted and treatable problems. Unfortunately more subtle problems related to yeast are usually ignored and not linked to patient's complaints. If a subject is not taught in medical school, it is assumed not to be real. Medical history proves this is a dangerous assumption.[62]

Also according to Dr. Hyman, "[Y]east overgrowth can be triggered by a number of things. These include a high-sugar, high-fat, low-fiber diet, impaired immunity, use of drugs like antibiotics, birth control pills, estrogen, and steroids like prednisone, and psychological stress."[63]

As far as diagnosis tests go, Dr. Hyman goes on to say:

> Many tests we use for diagnosis of yeast problems are not definitive or foolproof. It is often a diagnosis that must be made from a patient's story, symptoms, and physical findings on examination. Blood antibody levels for yeasts, stool tests, and organic acid urine tests (v) for yeast metabolites can be helpful if they come out positive but don't rule yeast out if they're negative.[64]

Symptoms of yeast vary, and Dr. Hyman recommends a systematic approach. Literature I have read on this subject all have very basic information for healing the body of this type of yeast. Two specific things they all required are: 1) a change in diet being essential to ridding the body of this fungal overgrowth, and 2) the immune system being rebuilt, and the beneficial flora or probiotics (as they are called today) being replenished on a regular basis in order to keep the bad bacteria (and *Candida* yeast) in balance.

On the *Candida* diet (which many call the diet for ridding the body of *Candida*), foods with sugar (including natural sugar) must be avoided: sugar (honey, maple syrup, agave, rice syrup, cane, etc.), refined grains of any kind, refined rice, refined foods (including cereal, pasta, etc.), and most fruit (except tart fruits like lemons, limes, and cranberries). Wines, beers, cheeses, and any other foods with sugars should be avoided as well.

Systemic *Candida* overgrowth is one of the most difficult of all bodily conditions to treat. Once a *Candida* infection spreads throughout the body, it is extremely hard to control. People can struggle for years attempting to cleanse their bodies, with the *Candida* diet, anti-fungal, probiotics (acidophilus), and the myriad products available in health food stores and on the Internet. There is no "magic pill" that cures *Candida.*

The typical, modern, Western diet of highly processed, cooked, acidic, and refined foods that are filled with all types of chemicals creates the perfect atmosphere for *Candida* to thrive. With *Candida* traveling throughout the body, the *Candida* can hide in places like joints, organs, and sinuses, and it is very difficult to remove. Many pharmaceutical drugs can provide temporary relief, but if the root of the problem isn't solved, then it will remain a constant problem. The drugs Diflucan and Eraxis have the side effect of possible liver damage, so these can result in a more challenging health situation. The root of the problem is the destruction of the beneficial bacteria in the body and the weakened immune system, along with an acidic environment. The beneficial bacteria need to be replenished and maintained on an ongoing basis. Most people today think is that it is normal to ingest chemicals and drugs. These are not food, and the body is affected dramatically whenever it is faced with the ingestion of chemicals and drugs.

From my own experience and in my opinion, pure food cures are the ones that will support the body in the most optimum way. Foods that help build the body's immune system and contribute to the healthy bacteria include onions, garlic, fermented vegetables, fermented coconut water or kefir, oregano oil, and coconut oil. A good cleanse that cleans out the intestinal tract is necessary to create healthy intestines. Seventy percent of our immune system is located in our intestines. If the intestinal tract is blocked with plaque, waste, debris, etc., the immune system is challenged. Also, most of our nutrients are absorbed through our intestinal wall. If the intestinal wall is blocked with plaque and waste, nutrients cannot get through.

A good intestinal cleanse can include high-fiber cleanses and/or colonics. A few *Candida* products can also help. Natalia Rose, a clinical nutritionist with whom I studied detoxification and cleansing in New York, suggested the product Candi Gone along with diet changes.

Dr. Hyman has his own plan. Here are some of his guidelines:

Overcoming Yeast Overgrowth

1. Address predisposing factors. Don't take antibiotics, steroids, or hormones unless absolutely medically necessary.

2. Eat a diet that doesn't feed yeast in the gut (low sugar and refined carbohydrates, and low mold and yeast in food).

3. Use probiotics to repopulate the gut with healthy bacteria.
4. Take antifungal herbs and medications when indicated.
5. Identify potential environmental toxic fungi and molds in your home or workplace.
6. Reduce stress.

The Yeast Control Eating Program

A simple five-day elimination of yeast and molds in your diet, followed by a challenge or binge of yeasty foods will often relieve and then trigger your symptoms…

Probiotics

Take at least 10 to 20 billion live organisms a day of lactobacillus and bifidobacter species. (vi) A special "yeast against yeast" probiotic called saccharomyces boulardii (vii) can be very safe and effective in controlling yeast.

Non-prescription Anti-fungal

Using antifungal therapies such as herbs and other naturally occurring compounds can be very helpful in controlling yeast. The dose for all of the following herbal remedies is generally two pills with meals, three times a day for two to three months. You might need less or more based on your response and symptoms. Sometimes these remedies can be combined for better effect. To find the right combinations and doses for you and identify quality products, consult with a qualified practitioner trained in functional medicine (www.functionalmedicine.org). Some of the best antifungal compounds include the following:

- Oregano—Oil of oregano has many antibacterial and antifungal properties.
- Garlic—Fresh, crushed garlic is a potent antimicrobial and immune booster.
- Citrus seed extract—The phytochemicals in citrus seeds have been found to have potent antimicrobial properties.
- Berberine—This potent yellow plant extract comes from goldenseal and barberry.
- Tannins—These are the astringent compounds found in tea and the bark of trees.
- Undecylenate—This chemical compound is a potent antifungal.
- Isatis tinctoria—This Chinese herb can be a useful adjunct to treating intestinal imbalances.
- Caprylic acid—This is another useful compound for treating yeast.[65]

It seems as if everyone who writes on this subject states that everyone is different, with different sensitivities and various dietary restrictions, so it is extremely important to be aware of that and learn to listen to your own body signals. Attempt to make your diet as sugar-free as possible, so it won't support or feed yeast. Think about keeping a food diary, so you can see accurately how you feel after consuming different foods in various situations. Try to make your home environment as free of mold or fungus as possible. Last but not least, relax and keep stress to a minimum.

Food for Stress Reduction

Foods that help our bodies cope with stress can be both a blessing and necessity.

One thing I have found to be quite helpful is the raw powder of the maca root. This powder originates in the Andes and has been identified as a super-food. (Super-foods are foods that have more nutrients in them than the foods we normally consume.) Maca root contains over 55 beneficial phyto-chemical nutrients. These chemicals assist our bodies with hormones, boosting mood and energy, and increasing stamina. Maca root can help rebuild weak immune systems and assist with re-mineralizing the body. Maca root is really helpful to the adrenal or suprarenal glands, which are weakened by stress. The adrenals are chiefly responsible for regulating our body's stress response. Common symptoms of adrenal fatigue include dark circles under the eyes, low blood sugar, lower back pain, knee weakness or pain, fatigue, cravings for sugar or salt, chronic infections, and lack of libido. The adrenal glands are very important for our immune system and proper thyroid function. Not many foods support and nurture the adrenal glands.

I buy raw, organic maca root powder and add it to my smoothies in the morning. The raw root is not processed over 118 degrees, and therefore it retains the live enzymes necessary to feed the cells of the body. You can purchase maca root powder at health food stores or online. Because our bodies can become allergic to anything that we consume (no matter how healthy it is) if we eat it constantly, I never eat a single ingredient every day. I eat certain foods four or five times a week, and keep a variety of seasonal fresh fruits and vegetables in my diet. Maca root does not have much flavor, so you can add it to many food combinations. It goes well with fruit or cacao smoothies.

I have always found working with my garden or food for the table to be a very relaxing and calming experience. When you are preparing food or taking your bath, light candles, put on nice music, and make it a wonderful, peaceful time. This can set a restful tone that can help relieve stress.

In addition to maca root, here are some other stress-reducing foods that you can add to your diet[66]:

Lentils, chickpeas, and quinoa are high in the B vitamins and have a calming effect on the body. The B vitamins can enhance your mood and help quell anxiety.

Papayas (yellow and orange fruits and vegetables) and red bell peppers have Vitamin A, Vitamin C, and folate, which enhance your mood, give you more energy, and repair cells damaged from stress.

Basil, arugula, and sunflower seeds all contain the nutrient folate, which helps with attaining a calmer mood.

Glutamine

Glutamine is an amino acid. I am including this amino acid because so many people are struggling with sugar and/or alcohol addiction and I thought this might be useful information.

Supplements have been studied to use as an aid in helping quell any kind of sugar/starch "craving."

Glutamine is the most abundant amino acid that is found primarily in your muscles. The human body cannot produce glutamine in sufficient quantities. Because of this, additional sources are sometimes needed. With diet and supplements, a person can supply the body with the additional glutamine that he or she requires. These supplements commonly come in a powder form, pill, or tablet. Some plant proteins are dietary sources of glutamine. A diet high in legumes is recommended for sufficient natural glutamine production.

> Glutamine enhances the intestine's ability to resist the invasion of harmful micro-organisms, as well as promoting cell reproduction and boosting the body's immune system. Glutamine is also one of the building blocks of glutathione, the body's primary antioxidant. It is often given to patients who have cancer, AIDS, trauma, burns and other infections, as it promotes the healing of wounds. Glutamine is a common supplemental treatment for peptic ulcers and in preventing aspirin-induced gastric lesions. It is often used as an oral rinse to reduce mouth sores usually associated with chemotherapy to treat cancer. It is also used to treat other cancer complications such as stomach irritation....
>
> **ALCOHOLISM AND SUGAR ADDICTION**
>
> Alcoholics and sugar addicts may find glutamine supplementation a way to ease the stomach pain and mental toxicity that comes when they stop consuming alcohol or sugar. It is thought that glutamine may reduce cravings.[67]

Hair Health

Hair can definitely be influenced by what we are consuming. I have heard about people who switched to a vegetarian diet and had a problem with hair loss. They were not getting the proper nutrition. In many cases hair loss is the result of a deficiency of Vitamin B and other nutrients. Lacking the right kind of essential fatty acids can also be part of the equation. A lack of Vitamin B6, folic acid, magnesium, sulfur, iodine, zinc, and multiple nutrients in the Vitamin B complex that the body needs in small amounts to function and stay healthy can result in hair thinning or hair loss. The combination of nutrients is what is important, including eating the right kind of proteins in the right amounts.

Foods rich in B vitamins are brewer's yeast, wheat germ, and lecithin. Beans are also high in protein and B vitamins. Vegetarians sometimes don't eat enough protein or get the right amount of Vitamin B, so it is important to make certain to eat enough protein and take whole-food based vitamins with Vitamin B complex to maintain health. Check to make sure the B9 is listed as folate and not folic acid (the synthetic version). Vegetarians can eat Nori seaweed and peanuts as sources of arachidonic acid, which is needed by the body to create a certain enzyme needed for fat metabolism. Meat eaters usually have an excess of this arachidonic acid (which is a third essential fatty acid) needed by the body but that the body does not provide.

There are many non–B vitamins and minerals that contribute to healthy hair. Zinc works in cell reproduction and hormone balance, affecting hair growth and taking care of the hair follicles. If the body is low in zinc, the hair follicles can become weak. Vegetarian foods heavy in zinc are nuts. Silica, the second-most-prevalent element on earth, which is found in the skin of potatoes, green and red peppers, cucumbers, bean sprouts, and raw oats, has been found to have numerous health benefits. With respect to hair loss, medical studies have found that adding organic silica to shampoo slows hair loss.

Vitamin E is another important element of healthy hair, having been shown to improve scalp circulation because of its anti-cellular aging and increased blood oxygenation properties. Avocados, kiwi fruit, nuts, seeds, and extra-virgin olive oil are good sources of Vitamin E.

Vitamin A's protection of hair follicles has been documented. Vitamin A can be found in carrots, spinach, and unrefined, cold-pressed seed oils, such as flax, walnut, and pumpkin.

Iodine is also essential to healthy hair. Iodine in whole-food form is found in sea vegetables (seaweed), cabbage, pine nuts, and millet.

Although it is best to get nutrients in a whole-food form, all of these vitamins and minerals can be found in supplement form. When buying supplements, look for organic, whole-food supplements. Your body can read whole foods much better than it can isolated chemical vitamins.

Essential fatty acids are another vital way of promoting healthy hair and skin. Make them a regular part of your diet, but remember to store them properly. Essential fatty acids can become rancid and therefore create free radicals in the body, which will foster aging and a weakened immune system. Essential oils should be stored in the refrigerator.

Because of this it is necessary to use fresh, cold-pressed oils and refrigerate them. Most people today don't get enough Omega 3 fatty acids. Fresh, cold-pressed flax seed oil could be one of the best remedies. It contains the right proportion of alpha-linolenic acid (Omega 3) and non-rancid linolenic acid, which is good because they work best as a combination. Some other essential fatty acid sources are walnuts, avocados, almonds, pecans, pumpkins, hazelnuts, pine nuts, sesame, olives, and their respective oils.

A good coffee bean grinder is a great way to add some of these nuts and seeds easily to foods. These grinders are about $20 and are well worth the investment. Mine is about 20 years old and I use it constantly. Just grind the fresh nuts or seeds in the grinder and sprinkle them on dishes the way you would a seasoning. My favorite is to add freshly ground flax seeds to salads, smoothies, casseroles, and soups. Don't buy already-ground flax seeds, because they will have lost some of the nutrients. You always want to have them freshly ground. Don't heat flax seeds; add them to the food after it is cool.

Health and the Peaceful Mind

True health is having true peace in our heart, mind, and soul. When we are totally at peace, we can have total health. What are you saying to yourself as you walk around all day and night? What thoughts are going through your mind? Every single thought is an affirmation. Whatever you are thinking about constantly is your affirmation. Change your affirmation to say nice things about yourself and your life. Don't focus on the negative; focus on the solution.

There is the child within you, in your heart and soul. Nurture your child within as you would your own child or other people's children.

Treat yourself with love and nurturing. Be patient with yourself. Give yourself a break. It is okay. Release old pains of the past; they do not serve you. Forgive yourself and others, and forget. It does not condone what others did, but it can free your mind from those negative thoughts that are only hurting you. Release them and set yourself free. Dwelling on things that happened in the past, keeps you in the past. What we think is a choice. Choose to live with joy and passion in the very present moment. You may see positive opportunities appear as soon as you start creating a positive, present mindset.

Iodine

One of the most important nutrients to support our health is iodine. It is an essential nutrient that supports the thyroid, our "master gland." It is central to all of our body's major functions. The thyroid influences our metabolism, digestion, energy, body temperature, skin, hair, sleep, mental acuity, nervous system, sexual organs, and hormonal system. In fact, it would be very difficult to find a system that is *not* influenced by the thyroid. Because of the thyroid's widespread effects, malfunction can significantly affect a person's life and poses a detriment to long-term health. It is difficult to have a healthy thyroid without iodine.

What foods contain iodine? Soil is pretty much depleted of this nutrient, and there are few foods that contain iodine. Up until 1980, bakeries added iodine to bread. After 1980, they switched from adding iodine and to adding potassium bromate. What does this mean? We have a certain amount of space for iodine in our thyroid. Our thyroid is located right in the bottom middle of the front of our neck. Our body can store about three months' worth of iodine in the cells. When we ingest potassium bromate, also called bromide, it acts like iodine and will take up the space in the thyroid reserved for iodine, and will actually prevent the body from absorbing the iodine it needs. The chlorine and fluoride that almost all municipal water companies in the United States put in water act the same way. These chemicals can all contribute to iodine deficiency.

Iodine is put in table salt. However, when it is exposed to oxygen, the iodine dissipates, so this is not really a reliable source. Also, table salt is actually refined sodium with added bicarbonates, chemicals, sugar, and preservatives. The minerals are removed, and the body reads this table salt as toxic chemicals.

Real sea salt is full of minerals and nutrients our body needs. True sea salt is rich in electrolytes, which help our body absorb water and feed our body on a deep cellular level. Most mineral salts have some iodine in them, in various amounts. Vitamin E and Vitamin D are important nutrients that can help the body absorb iodine.

Many doctors will only perform one inexpensive test for iodine deficiency. Frequently, it won't show a true picture of the deficiency. There are three more tests that will show a better picture of the iodine levels in your body, and you can ask your doctor for those tests.

There is also an inexpensive self-test you can perform at home to see if you have some iodine deficiency. Buy brown iodine at the pharmacy for a few dollars. Put some of the brown iodine on some soft tissue on the skin. Put it somewhere you won't be brushing with your clothing during the day, as it will stain. The clothing can also absorb the iodine and the test won't work.

Put the iodine on the skin and then wait. If your body absorbs it really quickly (within three or four hours), then your body is really low in iodine. If it is absorbed within 24 hours, you are low in iodine. The quicker the iodine is absorbed, the more iodine-deficient your body is.

Sea vegetables or seaweed is one of the few food sources of natural iodine that the body can readily absorb.

Vitamin E should be taken with an iodine supplement, in order to help with iodine absorption.[68] Add some sunflower seeds to this mixture for added nutrient-dense composition. Foods rich in Vitamin E are wheat germ, rice, oats, quinoa, broccoli, sprouts, spinach, dandelion greens, mint, almonds, and sunflower seeds.

In addition, you can buy liquid sea kelp and add it to water or smoothies. It really doesn't have a taste, so you can really add it to almost anything.

Iron

Vegetarians need to make certain that they have adequate iron required for optimum health. Iron is an essential mineral needed by the body to take oxygen to muscles and organs. Iron is also a necessary component for the regulation of cell growth and differentiation. Without iron, anemia can occur. I spent my whole life battling acute anemia (a result of a penicillin overdose when I was 2 years old). "A deficiency of iron limits oxygen delivery to cells, resulting in fatigue, poor work performance, and decreased immunity [1,5-6]. On the other hand, excess amounts of iron can result in toxicity and even death [7]."[70] It was not until I became a vegetarian that I was able to cure myself of the acute anemia.

Good sources of iron are asparagus, legumes (like lentils, lima beans, chickpeas, split peas, and red beans), dark green, leafy vegetables (like asparagus, spinach, Swiss chard, and beet greens), dried fruits (including prunes), and whole grains (such as whole wheat and bulgur). Iron is much better absorbed if Vitamin C or citrate is present, so eat foods high in Vitamin C when you eat foods with high iron counts. Foods rich in Vitamin C include citrus fruits, fresh berries, red bell peppers, tomatoes, and broccoli. There are also a few foods that can block or reduce the absorption of iron: tea, coffee, bran, dairy products, soy, and some spices (chili, rosemary, oregano, and cinnamon).

Recommended Dietary Allowances for Iron for Infants (7 to 12 Months), Children, and Adults[70]

Age	Males (mg/day)	Females (mg/day)	Pregnancy (mg/day)	Lactation (mg/day)
7 to 12 months	11	11	N/A	N/A
1 to 3 years	7	7	N/A	N/A
4 to 8 years	10	10	N/A	N/A
9 to 13 years	8	8	N/A	N/A
14 to 18 years	11	15	27	10
19 to 50 years	8	18	27	9
51+ years	8	8	N/A	N/A

Magnesium

"Q: What is the percentage of Americans with inadequate intakes of Magnesium from food based on estimated average requirements?

A: 56%"[71]

Magnesium deficiency is not specific to vegetarians or vegans. Magnesium is a trace mineral. It is necessary for hundreds of bodily functions. Magnesium deficiency has been linked to migraines, allergies, anxiety, asthma, attention deficit disorder, diabetes, calcification of soft tissue (including the heart valve), muscle cramps, osteoporosis, fibromyalgia, hearing loss, menstrual cramps, insomnia, irritability, trembling, twitching, and the list goes on. Magnesium deficiency can cause increased levels of adrenaline, which can cause feelings of anxiety. A Brown University study found magnesium extremely beneficial for children with acute asthma. Additionally, children with sensitive hearing may have low magnesium levels.

Two separate research teams comprised of researchers at the Harvard School of Public Health and Harvard Medical School published their findings on magnesium and reduced Type II diabetes risk in the January 2004 issue of the journal *Diabetes Care.*

Another factor for low magnesium may be the use of calcium supplements that don't include magnesium. "High calcium intakes can make magnesium deficiency worse," according to Forrest Nielsen.[72] He says additional magnesium can help. In an article on the USDA Agriculture Research Service website, Mr. Neilsen goes on to say: "The diets of many people do not contain enough magnesium for good health and sleep. In 1997, the United States Food and Nutrition Board set the recommended dietary allowance (or daily intake) for magnesium at 320 milligrams for women and 420 milligrams for men between ages 51 and 70."[73]

Foods that contain magnesium are beans, whole grains, nuts, and vegetables, especially green, leafy vegetables. Some tasty magnesium-rich food choices for children are baked potatoes, bananas, coconut milk, peas, peanut butter, bean burritos, and cashews. Caffeine and alcohol can cause a magnesium loss. Caffeine-rich foods include coffee, tea, some energy drinks and bars, and various types of soda.

MSG: A Hidden Danger in Processed and Restaurant Foods

Monosodium glutamate (MSG) is categorized as an excitotoxin. According to the book *Excitotoxins: The Taste that Kills*, by Russell Blaylock, MD, these excitotoxins will literally stimulate and excite neurons in the brain to death. This causes brain damage in various degrees, according to Dr. Blaylock, a neurosurgeon.

MSG was discovered in 1908 by Japanese chemist Kikunae Ikeda. Professor Ikeda was trying to isolate a chemical in seaweed: kombu, a flavor enhancer. What he came up with is glutamic acid combined with sodium molecule, which resulted in MSG. The component glutamate, or glutamic acid, is an excitatory amino acid neurotransmitter in the brain. These neurotransmitters in the brain are normal, but when there is an excess of them, they will be over-stimulated and die. These are extremely harmful to our brain health, according to Dr. Blaylock. Children and infants are even more vulnerable to this chemical. Today MSG is frequently made by a fermenting process using starch, sugar beets, sugar cane, or molasses.

Professor Kikunae Ikeda founded the Ajinomoto Company. His new product was a huge hit. MSG enhanced the flavor of food. The Japanese used it in many foods, including the food rations they gave to US prisoners of war. The US military was curious about why the American soldiers loved the food rations they received as prisoners of war of the Japanese. After the US military found out about the MSG, in 1948 the US Armed Forces met with the largest food companies in the United States and discussed how MSG could be added to various food products.

MSG has since been added to almost all processed foods as well as foods in almost all fast-food restaurants and other restaurants that you would not suspect. It has been huge for the food industry, because it actually makes you think that what you are eating tastes better. It works on the brain as a pleasure trigger. It can send pleasure impulses to the brain, until it kills that part of the brain. So, food that may normally taste a bit dull or bland may taste really great with MSG added to it. The diet food industry has really benefited from the use of MSG. Dr. Blaylock has tried for many years to educate people about these toxic addictives in our food supply. (His books are listed in the References.)

As of 2010, the FDA has no limit on how much of this can be added to food. Examples of foods that contain MSG are NutraSweet and aspartame. Theoretically, the long-term effects can be attention deficit/hyperactivity disorder (ADHD), autism, and other learning disabilities. In adults, conditions such as Parkinson's, Alzheimer's, and Lou Gehrig's diseases, multiple sclerosis, auto-immune disease, sleep disorders, migraines, and the inability to lose weight may be linked to excitotoxin damage. Over the years, a greater and greater amount of MSG has been added to foods.

Hydrolyzed Proteins

Hydrolyzed proteins are flavor enhancers. Hydrolyzed proteins are proteins that have been chemically broken down into amino acids. When these proteins are chemically broken down (during the body's digestive process), the result can be the creation of free glutamate, which joins with free sodium (in the body) to form MSG. This does not have to be put on an ingredient label like MSG does when it is added in full form. Free glutamate can cause the body to react like it has had a stimulating drug given to the nervous system. It can affect insulin metabolism and create escessive insulin secretion by the pancreas. Some common symptoms of having this reaction are anxiety attacks, asthma-like symptoms, attention deficit disorder, burning sensations, carpal tunnel syndrome, chest pains, depression, diarrhea, disorientation and confusion, dizziness, drowsiness, fatigue, flushing, gastric distress, headaches and migraines, hyperactivity in children, infertility and other endocrine problems, insomnia, irregular or rapid heart beat, joint pain, mood swings, mouth lesions, nausea and vomiting, numbness (such as fingertips), seizures, shortness of breath, simple skin rash, slurred speech, stomach-aches, tremors, and weakness.

Here is a partial list of hidden sources of MSG that Dr. Blaylock includes in his book *Excitotoxins: The Taste that Kills*. (For more information, his book is a great source.) Some of the ingredients aren't MSG when they are put into the food, but when they touch saliva, they create MSG. Many of these look just like "normal" food ingredients. Many of them are added to alternative meat products that are sold as vegetarian foods. That is why buying whole, fresh foods and making your food yourself are becoming more and more important for health.

Additives that always contain MSG:

Monosodium glutamate
Hydrolyzed vegetable protein
Hydrolyzed protein
Hydrolyzed plant protein
Plant protein extract
Yeast extract
Textured protein
Autolyzed yeast
Hydrolyzed oat flour

Additives that frequently contain MSG:

Malt flavoring and/or extract
Bouillon
Broth
Stock
Flavoring
Natural flavoring
Seasoning
Spices

Additives that may contain MSG or excitotoxins:

Enzymes
Soy protein concentrate or isolate
Whey protein concentrate

Probiotics and Our Immune System

What is our immune system and how do we support it? Over 70 percent of our immune system is located in our digestive tract. The major part of the immune system is comprised of a micro flora beneficial bacterium. You may hear these micro flora beneficial bacteria called probiotics. Probiotics, according to the World Health Organization and the Food and Agriculture Organization of the United States, are "live microorganisms, which, when administered in adequate amounts, confer a health benefit to the host."[74] "Friendly bacteria" is another name for probiotics. Why are probiotics important? "Friendly or positive bacteria are vital to proper development of the immune system, to protection against microorganisms that could cause disease, and to the digestion and absorption of food and nutrients."[75] With the widespread use of antibiotics, the beneficial bacteria (also called beneficial flora) in our bodies have become compromised. Antibiotics wipe out all bacteria, good and bad. Good bacteria keep bad bacteria in balance. If we don't have any good bacteria (or flora) in our system to support our immune system, then our immune system is compromised. The addition of probiotic food is vital to the health and strength of the immune system.

Our lives have become saturated with antibiotics. Antibiotics are in our water supply because of people disposing of medicines and using the restroom, as well as run-off from farms. Farms are the number-one purchaser of antibiotics. Many farm animals are given antibiotics on a regular basis. Any time you use an antibacterial, germ-killing gel (hand sanitizer) or soap, it is like taking an antibiotic. The antibacterial from the soap or sanitizer is absorbed right into the skin, like the medicine on a skin patch. It goes right into the blood stream. This can kill the beneficial bacteria in the body, just like taking an oral antibiotic capsule or pill. Because of the widespread saturation of antibiotics in our lives, it is important to replenish these beneficial bacteria on a regular, ongoing basis. Try making some form of these probiotic foods a part of your daily diet: garlic; onions; raw, unprocessed apple cider vinegar; raw, unprocessed soy sauce; coconut yogurts; some cottage cheese; miso; tempeh; some coconut products; and fermented foods.

Processed Foods, Fast Foods, and Refined Carbohydrates: Beware!

It is important to realize that many vegan or vegetarian foods are actually not healthy foods. Packaged foods, fast foods, processed foods, bakery foods, restaurant foods, and some grocery store foods can contain refined grains, refined salt, refined sugars, trans fats, chemicals, and other extremely unhealthy ingredients. Just because a food is vegetarian or vegan does not necessarily mean that the food is healthy. Many ingredient labels may have ingredients listed (or even *not* listed) that can leave you wondering what is really in the food. Many keep ingredients unknown. You may never know what is in a food or body care product. A product called "natural" may be made completely of chemically derived ingredients. The fact that the ingredient or product can be completely composed of chemicals and still be labeled "natural" can be very misleading.

Many foods that vegetarians eat may be high in sugar and/or refined or processed flours (carbohydrates), which the body reads as sugar. The body will read these nutrient empty and fiberless foods as sugar, which then causes blood sugar to spike. This makes the body work hard to bring the blood sugar level into balance. When the body is constantly working to keep blood sugar regulated, it can become exhausted and unable to regulate it. This can result in diabetes. In order for the body to process nutrient-empty (refined) food, it must pull nutrients from the body. This is one of the main reasons carbohydrates have a reputation as being unhealthy. It is not the carbohydrate that is unhealthy; it is the *type of* carbohydrate that is unhealthy. Carbohydrates are actually the body's preferred fuel. Whole grains that are nutrient-dense and fiber-dense, are nutritious, and can give your body the fuel it needs.

Refined carbohydrates and unrefined carbohydrates are not converted into glucose in the same way. Unrefined carbohydrates (for example, legumes, whole grains, and vegetables) are fiber-rich and take longer to digest. This will not put additional pressure on the pancreas to produce insulin in an unhealthy way. Refined carbohydrates (for example, white, refined flour, pasta, and bakery goods) have no or little fiber, and they convert to glucose quickly and put pressure on the pancreas to make insulin to get it under control. If too many of these refined carbohydrates are eaten on a continual basis, shooting up blood sugar levels, this will stress the pancreas and eventually the body will have trouble making insulin. The body will turn the excess glucose produced by the body into fat. This can result in excessive weight and obesity. A body with too much fat will also have problems, because the body will start ignoring the signal to take glucose from the blood. The spiking of blood sugar with refined and empty food can also result in cravings. When the body is not getting the nutrients it needs, it will start begging for the nutrients. When the body is fed with nutrient-dense food, it gets the nutrients it needs and there shouldn't be cravings.

Whole-grain carbohydrates should be a major part of a well-balanced vegetarian diet. When looking at a package that says "whole wheat" or "whole grain" on the front of the package, read the ingredient list and make sure it says "whole" before every grain listed. Packaging can be very deceiving and misleading. If a food is enriched or refined, it has had the nutrients and fiber removed. If the ingredient list contains just the name of the grain, then it is *not* whole grain. Make sure all the grains listed on the ingredient list are *whole grain.*

The front of the package may indicate that a product contains a certain ingredient, but then, when you look on the ingredient list, a totally different ingredient may be included as the major part of the product—with a miniscule part of the product being the one advertised on the front of the package. This is legal and very misleading. One pasta product, for example, says it's "quinoa pasta," but according to the ingredients it is mainly corn.

Be a savvy consumer. Now that you are aware of this, ask the owner or the person in charge of the bakery you patronize if the product is "all" whole grain, or look on the package and check the ingredients for yourself. Also remember that ingredients can change periodically in products. Even though you may have bought a product previously, it never hurts to check the ingredient list periodically.

Protein

What about protein? This is a common question people ask when I say I am a vegetarian. Protein is essential for maintaining healthy sugar levels in the blood, especially when eating carbohydrates. Protein is made up of amino acids, and is a crucial part of building and maintaining cells and tissues. The body uses amino acids to make hemoglobin and insulin, which are necessary for being healthy. People have been obsessed with protein for centuries. Because this subject is so controversial and almost always the first question out of anyone's mouth when hearing someone is a vegetarian, I decided to cover protein at great length.

I will begin back at the beginning of the 20th century, with Russel Henry Chittenden, the father of biochemistry, who wrote *Physiological Economy in Nutrition*. Chittenden was disturbed by his observation of physicians recommending high-protein diets of 135 grams a day. He thought this was wrong and set out to test this dietary theory, because there was not one "spec of science"[78] to support that high-protein-diet recommendation. Chittenden began by doing a study on himself using a low-protein diet. In that study, he lost weight, had more energy, got rid of his arthritic joint pain, and was, in his opinion, healthier than he had been on a high-protein diet. This study being a success, he began testing his Yale colleagues, Yale students, and finally Yale athletes. In his study, "Chittenden's data proved that even without a large protein intake, individuals could maintain their health and fitness.... The results are presented as scientific facts, and the conclusions they justify are self-evident."[77]

In fact, in Chittenden's study, every single person, which included Chittenden himself, five Yale faculty members, 18 hospital Corp of U.S. Army, and eight Yale student-athletes (he had the student-athletes on 64 grams of protein a day), on this low-protein diet had more energy, felt better, and actually increased their performance ability by over 35 percent. The study was well documented at the time, including dietary history and urine analysis. "Chittenden in 1904 concluded that 35–50 g of protein a day was adequate for adults, and individuals could maintain their health and fitness on this amount. Studies over the past century have consistently confirmed Professor Chittenden's findings."[78]

Some studies say people that should also be eating for their blood type. Dr. Peter J. D'Adamo and Catherine Whitney's book on the connection between blood type, diet, and health, *Eat Right 4 Your Type,* expands on this. My blood type is O, as is my daughter's. The book says that "O blood types are meant to thrive best on a high protein (red meat) and low carbohydrate diet."[79] I have been vegetarian for 25 years and so has my daughter. We seem to do quite well on a vegetarian diet, but we do make sure we consume enough high-protein-rich plant foods like beans, lentils, nuts, seeds, whole grain rice, and quinoa, and have a good amount of healthy fats in our diet. The authors also say that A blood types are supposed to be vegetarian (high carbohydrate and low fat); B blood types should eat dairy, meat, fish, grains, vegetables, and fruit; and AB blood types should consume mostly vegetarian food, with moderate meat and dairy. In the book the authors list various foods that are good, better, best, or worse for each blood type.[80] It is up to you to decide if this theory is right for you.

Many athletes today are extremely concerned about protein. The Vegetarian Resource Group offers some good information concerning protein. Congruent with Chittenden's results, according to the Vegetarian Resource Group:

> Vegans are bombarded with questions about where they get their protein. Athletes used to eat thick steaks before competition because they thought it would improve their performance. Protein supplements are sold at health food stores. This concern about protein is misplaced. Although protein is certainly an essential nutrient which plays many key roles in the way our bodies function, we do not need huge quantities of it. In reality, we need small amounts of protein. Only one calorie out of every ten we take in needs to come from protein. Athletes do not need much more protein than the general public.[78]

Many athletes today are filling their bodies with protein-rich food, thinking it will make them stronger and their muscles bigger. In an *AARP* article, tennis athlete Martina Navratilova says:

> On days that I work out, I'll have a little protein with some carbs after exercising. This combo speeds up the manufacture of new glycogen (the carbohydrate that is stored in muscle and supplies energy) and elevates key hormones in the body that are involved in muscle repair and growth. In addition, the snack amplifies the fuel I get from carbs.[82]

This fits with what I have read from other top athletes, like Brendan Brazier, two-time Canadian 50 K ultra-marathon champion. He thinks recovery time from working out is really what is the most critical when you are an athlete. He lives and thrives on a 100-percent plant-based diet. Many vegetarian proteins are a combination of carbohydrates and protein. You can find some great information about protein and the vegan athlete on the vegan athlete websites listed in the Resources. Our bodies are all different and our blood types are different, and you need to find what works best for you.

Protein myths have been around for over a century, but when the book *Diet for a Small Planet* by Frances Moore Lappe was published in 1971, it started a revolution that has impacted millions of people's lives ever since. According to Dr. John McDougall, Frances Moore Lappe did not understand the scientific research on human protein needs and the sufficiency of plant-based foods. Therefore she wrote that plants contained "incomplete proteins" with inadequate amounts of specific essential amino acids for them to meet the dietary needs of people. She emphasized combining vegetable-based foods in order to obtain the complete amino acid complexes needed for optimum health as compared to animal protein. Dr. John McDougall says that plant combining "is unnecessary and implies that it is difficult to obtain 'complete' protein from vegetables without detailed nutritional knowledge. Because of her complicated and incorrect ideas people are frightened away from vegetable-based diets."[83]

Thankfully those myths are slowly but surely being dismissed as untrue. The Cleveland Clinic, which has been ranked by *U.S. News & World Report* as the nation's number-one heart care program in the country for 17 consecutive years[84], addresses the vegetarian diet and this situation. It says: "The American Dietetic Association (ADA) recently revised their position statement on vegetarian diets. Changing their stance from previous publications, the ADA now agrees that well-planned vegetarian diets are a healthy nutritionally adequate dietary practice for all stages of life." In their section on the vegetarian diet, they state:

> Studies have shown that you can get the recommended amount of essential amino acids when you consume a variety of plant foods throughout the day. Complementing proteins at meals is no longer believed to be necessary to meet total protein requirements. To ensure adequate protein intake, consume a variety of plant foods daily. Good sources of plant protein include beans (e.g. kidney, navy, edamame, black) tofu, nuts and seeds. Whole grains and vegetables are also good sources of protein.[85]

Dr. Andrew Weil, a prominent doctor in the health field, also addressed this subject: "You may have heard that vegetable sources of protein are incomplete and become complete only when correctly combined. Research has discredited that notion so you don't have to worry that you won't get enough usable protein if you don't put together some magical combination of foods at each meal."[86]

He goes on to say:

> Whether or not you're a vegetarian, I recommend that you divide your daily calories as follows: 40 to 50 percent from carbohydrates (including vegetables, fruit, whole grains, starchy roots and tubers, and legumes), 30 percent from fat, and 20 to 30 percent from protein, which amounts to between 100 and 150 grams on a 2,000 calorie-a-day diet.[87]

Dr. Weil, then, actually recommends more protein than Dr. Chittenden. Take into account that Dr. Chittenden was probably using "meat" protein as a good portion of his diet study. So, the type of protein may vary from person to person. In my opinion, you have to decide what type and amount of protein works best for you.

Back to protein combining. Dennis Gordon, MEd, RD, voices the same opinion as Dr. Weil and Dr. McDougall. In the article "Vegetable Proteins Can Stand Alone," Gordon wrote:

> Complementing proteins is not necessary with

> vegetable proteins. The myth that vegetable source proteins need to be complemented is similar to the myths that persist about sugar making one's blood glucose go up faster than starch does. These myths have great staying power despite their being no evidence to support them and plenty to refute them.[88]

Reed Mangels, PhD, RD, also has spoken about protein combining:

> It is very easy for a vegan diet to meet the recommendations for protein, as long as calorie intake is adequate. Strict protein combining is not necessary; it is more important to eat a varied diet throughout the day.... The RDA recommends that we take in 0.8 grams of protein for every kilogram that we weigh (or about 0.36 grams of protein per pound that we weigh).... This recommendation includes a generous safety factor for most people.... To meet protein recommendations, the typical adult male vegan needs only 2.5 to 2.9 grams of protein per 100 calories and the typical adult female vegan needs only 2.1 to 2.4 grams of protein per 100 calories. These recommendations can be easily met from vegan sources.[89]

Protein myths have been around for almost a century, but beans, seeds, leafy greens, legumes, grains, eggs, and dairy are all sources of protein. In fact, leafy greens are among the best sources of protein. For example, 45 percent of spinach is protein.

Nuts and Seeds

Nuts and seeds are perfect foods, because they are a combination of protein, fat, and carbohydrate.

Pine nuts (pignoli) are wonderful to add to a meal-replacement or protein drink, to use if you are making a smoothie, or to have as a snack. Pine nuts are nature's only source of pinolenic acid, which helps diminish your appetite. Pine nuts have the highest concentration of oleic acid, a mono-unsaturated fat that aids the liver in eliminating harmful triglycerides from our body, which helps protect our heart. Pine nuts are also packed with 3mg of iron per 1-ounce serving and are rich in Vitamin B1 and Vitamin B3, manganese, copper, magnesium, molybdenum, and zinc, as well as being a source of Vitamin B2, Vitamin E, and potassium. There are over 29 varieties of pine nuts. Most of the pine nuts in US grocery stores are from trees in China, Mexico, and Korea. All pine nuts are nutritious, but Mediterranean pine nuts (seeds from the Stone Pine [pinus pinea] or Umbrella Pine) or pignolia are more nutrient-dense. This variety of pine tree is native to Portugal, Spain, and Italy. Mediterranean pine nuts are lower in calories, have a great ratio of Omega 3 to Omega 6 essentail fatty acids, have a higher level of phytosterols (which are known for lowering cholesterol), and have a higher protein content than the other varieties of pine nut. Mediterranean pine nuts are long with an even diameter.

Hemp seeds are actually nuts. They contain significant amounts of Omega 3s and Omega 6s, as well as protein. They also contain significant amounts of Vitamin E, which is important for the thyroid gland. Hemp seeds are seen as an excellent food source because of their great combination of high-quality oil (44%) or "good" fat, protein (33%), and fiber (12%). Hemp protein contains all the complex amino acid proteins and is extremely similar to the type of protein in animal foods. It has a wonderful digestibility and appears to be free of the anti-nutrients found in soy. Hemp seeds or nuts deliver a good source of readily absorbable, nutrient-dense protein that can be readily utilized by the body.[90]

Almonds are actually seeds. They are a powerhouse of nutrients, including manganese, magnesium, copper, Vitamin B2, and phosphorus, and are a great source of protein and fiber. One-fourth cup of almonds has 12 grams of protein. That is more than two times the amount of protein in one egg. One problem with almonds is that they contain 1,800 more Omega 6s than Omega 3s. This can seriously throw off the balance of Omega 3s to Omega 6s in the body. Be mindful of this. Because of the balance of Omega 6s to Omega 3s, I tend to use more whole-grain rice milk these days than the almond milk I used to make when I started consuming and making non-dairy milk.

English walnuts (types of walnuts are different) are especially good for the vegetarian diet. They are high in protein; are a very good source of manganese, copper, tryptophan, and Omega 3s and Omega 6s; and have a fairly good ratio of Omega 3s to Omega 6s (4 Omega 6s to 1 Omega 3) and only 8% saturated fat.

Cashews are a very good source of copper, magnesium, tryptophan, and phosphorus. Copper is necessary to maintain healthy bones as well as connective tissues. Cashews have 117 Omega 6s to 1 Omega 3, and have 12.5% saturated fat. I love cashews, but I try to combine them with other nuts and seeds when I eat them to help balance out the omegas and saturated fats. Since I am an O blood type, which is supposed to be a protein/meat eater type, I probably handle saturated fats like these better than people with a different blood type.

Pumpkin seeds are a good source of protein and fiber, as well as minerals, including zinc, iron, magnesium, phosphorus, potassium, copper, and manganese. Pumpkin seeds have 117 Omega 6s to 1 Omega 3 and have a saturated fat content of 14%. The interesting thing about pumpkin seeds is that they are terrific in helping the body get rid of parasites. I use them on a regular basis when feeding the wild animals I rehabilitate. (I am a licensed certified wildlife rehabilitator.) I give the animals freshly ground (meaning that I grind them the moment I am using them) pumpkin seeds in their food, and it is amazing to me how many tape worms and other types of parasites come out in their bowel movements. Because of this, I use pumpkin seeds frequently, in a freshly ground form, in my own foods.

Nuts and seeds contain delicate polyunsaturated fatty acids that can become rancid shortly after being shelled. Nuts that come from tropical climates can contain high levels of fungal mycotoxins, which result from improper storage.

Almost all nuts and seeds also contain certain compounds that include enzyme inhibitors and phytic acid. Store nuts and seeds in a tightly sealed container (preferably glass) in the refrigerator. If you are going to eat them within a few days, soak them in a glass or steel bowl for 12 to 18 hours in non-chlorinated water and a little bit of whole sea salt. Then you can dehydrate or roast them in the oven at a low temperature, if you want them to be drier. Doing so will make them more digestible and help diminish some or most of the phytic acid and enzyme inhibitors. Look for products that are sprouted or say that they have been soaked. You may want to have your physician check your mineral levels, if you have a diet high in these foods.

Protein Supplements

There are some really good vegetarian protein supplements. If you are going to use a protein supplement, I recommend using one that contains protein that is organic, vegan, gluten-free, raw, and whole-grain. Sometimes people feel they are just not getting enough food, protein, or sustenance; they probably need some concentrated nutrients from protein and carbohydrates, along with some good fat. When the body is getting the combination of protein, carbohydrates, and fat from nutrient-dense, whole food full of live enzymes, the body can feel nutritionally satisfied. Studies have shown that after an intense workout, it is helpful to replenish the glycogen by having some carbohydrates combined with some protein, which appears to really support muscle. The fat tells the body how to utilize the protein and carbohydrates. Sometimes when people say they need protein, their body really needs good fat. When I use a meal replacement or protein powder, I add about a tablespoon of a fat to the mixture (usually coconut oil or flax seed oil, or a combination of both).

I list a few really good, certified organic protein supplements in the Resources. Protein supplements made from sprouted seeds, nuts, whole grains, whole-grain rice, hemp seeds, legumes, peas, and beans are some of my favorites. When buying protein supplements, just be careful to check that they aren't mystery protein; read the ingredient list very carefully. Anything that simply says "protein" could be ground-up leftovers from meat-packing plants, which can be the hair, nails, and hooves, as well as other parts, of the dead animals.

Be careful which protein powders or supplements you buy. Many of the protein supplements in 15 drinks that *Consumer Reports* tested contained levels of heavy toxic metals. Here is an excerpt from the report:

> ...[O]ur investigation, including tests at an outside laboratory of 15 protein drinks, a review of government documents, and interviews with health and fitness experts and consumers, found most people already get enough protein, and there are far better and cheaper ways to add more if it's needed. Some protein drinks can even pose health risks, including exposure to potentially harmful heavy metals,

> if consumed frequently. All drinks in our tests had at least one sample containing one or more of the following contaminants: arsenic, cadmium, lead, and mercury. Those metals can have toxic effects on several organs in the body.[91]

Again, read the ingredients carefully and buy ones that contain only organic, whole vegetarian food.

Marketing for these high-protein drinks is sharp, savvy, and targeted to body builders, athletes, Baby Boomers, and pregnant women. The advertising can say the drinks build muscle or help shed unwanted pounds. People have the idea that if they eat more protein, their bodies will build more muscle. Lifting weights and exercising are what build muscles.

Whey

Whey protein is commonly added to protein powders or body builder protein drinks. Whey protein isolate is dairy and considered vegetarian. Whey protein is a naturally occurring substance that is derived from milk. Whey is separated from the curds during the cheese-making process. It is usually refined into a powder. The powder can then be mixed with beverages such as juice. Since whey is derived from milk and has some lactose in it, people not capable of digesting lactose can have allergic reactions such as sneezing, itching, and rashes after ingesting whey. Whey protein is widely marketed in many products to athletes, seniors, teenagers, etc. for many reasons, including meal replacement, weight loss, and body building. Many people ingest excessive amounts of whey protein. They may consume these whey drinks or supplements and not be aware of the amount of whey protein or accumulative protein that they are ingesting.

Excess protein is damaging to the body. Excess whey protein can cause ketosis, which is, according to Northwestern University Sciences, a state of starvation when the body produces ketones.[92] Ketones are strenuous on the kidneys and can impair cognitive function. Ketosis can also cause dehydration, especially if you are losing a lot of water by exercising. Northwestern University Health Sciences further reports that ketosis can also cause insulin resistance and glucose intolerance, two primary factors of coronary artery disease. The American Council on Exercise reported that large amounts of whey protein can be stored as a form of fat. Studies have shown that whey protein can also stress the liver and kidneys, because the majority of protein is broken down by the liver and kidneys.

According to a study in the *International Journal of Sport Nutrition and Exercise Metabolism*, protein ingestion of less than 2.8 grams per kg body-weight does not harm renal function in athletes. The American Diabetes Association recommends that diabetic individuals consume only the recommended daily amount or less than that. Liver and kidney disease patients should ensure that their whey protein intake is closely monitored to avoid complications. The National Institutes of Health recommends a moderate protein diet even for those who do not have a history of kidney stones. Excessive whey protein intake can result in kidney stones or calcium deposits in the kidney, which can be very harmful if untreated.[93]

Add this to the results of the studies from Northwestern University, and you have some pretty good reasons to be very cautious about using whey protein powders on a regular basis.

Soy

Soy protein is a complete protein, but can be very hard to digest. The Chinese did not eat unfermented soybeans, because they contained quantities of natural toxins or "anti-nutrients," as well as being high in phytic acid. What this means is that ingestion of soy can keep the body from absorbing other nutrients, like calcium, magnesium, copper, iron, zinc, and particularly protein. In China, soy was not used as a "food" until fermentation techniques were discovered in the Chou Dynasty. When soy is fermented, as in miso, tempeh, or soy sauce, the soy nutrients are more digestible and easier to absorb.

"Soy can cause serious gastric distress, pancreatic distress, which can include cancer, and deficiencies in amino acid uptake."[94] "Soy also contains goitrogens—substances that are known to depress thyroid function."[95] Soy isolate is a food to avoid completely. The processing of this food is done mostly in aluminum tanks that leach high levels of aluminum into the food. Then MSG, flavorings, preservatives, sweeteners, and/or synthetic chemicals are frequently added in order to help get rid of the "beany" taste and to add a more "meaty" flavor. In animal experiments, the test animals used developed enlarged organs, particularly the thyroid and the pancreas.

Most soy on the market today is from genetically modified (GM) seed: 91 percent of soybeans planted in the United States and rapidly growing throughout the world, according to Natural News newsletter.[96] "More than 95 per cent of GM soy (and 75 per cent of other GM crops) is engineered to tolerate glyphosate herbicide, the most common formulation of which is Roundup."[97] This is just one more reason why I don't eat soy anymore, if I can possibly avoid it. I highly recommend reading more about glyphosate herbicide, if you are eating non-certified organic foods. (There are some reading materials listed in the Resources.)

Soy is not only sold as a food, but beware that soy is added to tortillas, breads, fake meats, and many other foods for the "health" benefit. Really it is just cheap filler and, in my opinion, used with the excuse that it is a "health" benefit. Again, read ingredient lists carefully. In an article by health and nutrition expert Dr. Joseph Mercola, "Learn the Truth About Soy: Just How Much Soy Do Asians Eat?" he says that the advertising industry has really misled the public about the safety and health benefits of soy, as well as the widespread use of it in the Asian diet. He states: "A study of the history of soy use in Asia shows that the poor used it during times of extreme food shortage, and only then the soybeans were carefully prepared (e.g. by lengthy fermentation) to destroy the soy toxins."[98]

He goes on to say that soy is not fed to infants and that there was a study done theorizing this method of food, but that it was not saying that this was an optimum way to feed an infant. Here is a quote concerning this study to which he refers:

> The whole purpose of this report was to comment on the possible use of soymilk to address the problem of feeding those infants without sufficient maternal milk in a country where cow's milk was not native. He again noted that although a weak soy milk or "tofu chiang" was "sold hot in Peking by street vendors and was taken by old people in place of tea", that "contrary to Western notions" it was not usual to feed soy milk to infants.[99]

Just be aware that there is a billion-dollar industry that supports and advertises soy as a health answer to many health situations. Soy is frequently touted as being the answer to women's menopause problems, heart disease, and weight problems, as well as a great protein source. When you are aware of this fact, you can be savvier when you are reading food labels or product packages that refer to soy having health benefits. Consider this: "Foods that contain at least 6.25 grams of soy, less than 3 grams of fat, less than 1 gram of saturated fat, and less than 20 milligrams of cholesterol can legally display an FDA-approved statement about soy's role in helping to lower heart disease risk."[100]

To address these health claims, in the year 2000, two FDA employees, Daniel Doerge and Daniel Sheehan, were worried enough about the danger of soy as food that they wrote a controversial letter of protest to their own employer, protesting the positive health claims for soy that the FDA was approving at the time.[101] They wrote:

> ...[T]here is abundant evidence that some of the isoflavones found in soy, including genistein and equol, a metabolize of daidzen, demonstrate toxicity in estrogen sensitive tissues and in the thyroid. This is true for a number of species, including humans. Additionally, isoflavones are inhibitors of the thyroid peroxidase which makes T3 and T4. Inhibition can be expected to generate thyroid abnormalities, including goiter and autoimmune thyroiditis. There exists a significant body of animal data that demonstrates goitrogenic and even carcinogenic effects of soy products. Moreover, there are significant reports of goitrogenic effects from soy consumption in human infants.[102]

Think carefully about the effects that soy can have on the thyroid (one of our master glands, which affect almost all aspects of our health) and estrogen. So many doctors and nutritionists are soy proponents. Be careful, and research this yourself if you are concerned.

One of the reasons soy is touted as a great health food is because it is said to help with menopause hormone imbalances. This is one of the reasons why so many doctors and older women were so happy to embrace it. Soy and soy-based products contain isoflavones or phytoestrogens, which are plant-based estrogens. Soy is not the only food that contains phytoestrogens. There are other, less controversial, and more digestible foods with phytoestrogens that can be consumed. (For more information on phytoestrogens, see the "Phytoestrogens and Breast Cancer—Fact Sheet #01" entry in the Resources.)

Furthermore, as far as soy isoflavones are concerned, for

> "men, eating soy isoflavones can significantly reduce testicular function and lower luteinizing hormone (LH) production, which is what signals the testicles to work. A high soy intake and potentially lower level of LH increases the probability of estrogen dominance in men, contributing to hair loss, swollen and cancerous prostates, and insulin resistance. Dorris Rapp, MD, a leading pediatric allergist, asserts that environmental and food estrogens are responsible for the worldwide reduction in male fertility."[103]

It is also important to be aware that soy can create allergic reactions. "In 1986, Stuart Berger, MD, placed soy among the seven top allergens-one of the "sinister seven."

Finally, let's address soy isolate. It is found in a huge variety of "vegan" foods. What is soy isolate?

> Soy protein isolate is actually the byproduct of soybean oil processing. To make soy protein isolate, soybeans (practically all the soybeans used to make soy protein are of the Monsanto variety, by the way) are first dehulled, then tempered and crushed to extract oil. The leftover soy "chunks" (which still contain fiber, water, some fat, and other carbohydrates) then undergo another extraction process that involves hexane—a neurotoxin that is also a substantial component in gasoline. The next step involves soaking these chunks in a chemical mixture (which commonly contains ammonia and hydrochloric acid) to help concen-

> trate protein levels and achieve a sponge-like texture. Finally, the mixture is then spray-dried.[104]

When processing standard soybeans, the result of the conversion to soy protein isolate is from a regular, standard soybean that is 40 percent protein to the soy protein isolate, which is usually about 95 percent protein.

Soy protein isolate is only made in factories. In fact, soy protein can only be made in factories. Healthy, whole foods should be able to be made in a kitchen. You can grind your own almond flour at home from almonds. You can make your own seitan (wheat meat) at home. You can make your own rice milk or hemp milk at home with a blender and some whole-food ingredients. You have to take into account that the only way to make soy protein isolate is by using extremely flammable and hazardous chemicals, like hexane, and extreme temperatures that you could not possibly obtain in a kitchen setting.

"By the way—organic soy protein isolate does not utilize hexane in any step of the process. The folks at The Cornucopia Institute has created a list to let you know which protein bars and soy burgers utilize hexane-extracted soy protein isolates (and which don't)."[105] http://www.cornucopia.org/hexane-guides/hexane_guide_bars.html

As I researched soy, I came to seriously reconsider its use. When I first became a vegetarian, I used soy for many things. Soy milk, soy beans, etc. were foods that I thought I should use. I learn something new every day. No one knows everything, so be open to new information.

I found soy foods that were vegetarian-style alternative meats that worked really well as transition foods from a meat-based diet. Some of them didn't taste very good and were a huge waste of money, but a few were pretty good. I always looked for organic ones, but many of them were not organic. I slowly weaned myself off of them. There are many more choices today that are organic and taste much better than what was available in 1988. As I have learned more about soy, I now don't eat it if possible. I do, however, use organic fermented soy sauces. I also use organic miso and tempeh occasionally. There are alternative organic misos now that are made with brown rice, garbanzo beans, and barley, and they taste terrific. I buy these instead of the soy variety. I read a very long, five-part article online recently. Here's an excerpt:

> There's also a serious connection between soy and

> cancer in adults—especially breast cancer. That's why the governments of Israel, the UK, France and New Zealand are already cracking down hard on soy....
>
> In sad contrast, 60 percent of the refined foods in U.S. supermarkets now contain soy. Worse, soy use may double in the next few years because (last I heard) the out-of-touch medicrats in the FDA hierarchy are considering allowing manufacturers of cereal, energy bars, fake milk, fake yogurt, etc., to claim that "soy prevents cancer." It doesn't....
>
> P.S.: Soy sauce is fine. Unlike soy milk, it's perfectly safe because it's fermented, which changes its molecular structure. Miso, natto and tempeh are also OK, but avoid tofu.[106]

In conclusion, if you are going to buy soy, buy certified organic soy, because it won't be from genetically modified seeds. Buy sprouted and/or fermented soy for a more digestible and less harmful soy protein, and avoid soy isolates.

Beans

Beans, including black beans, garbanzo beans (also known as chickpeas), pinto beans, and kidney beans, are another great source of protein, fiber, and anti-oxidants. Beans are relatively inexpensive and easy to store in a dry, cool place for a fairly long time.

Beans are a leading food rich in fiber. The fiber in beans has been shown to help lower cholesterol by binding with bile acids, which are used in making cholesterol. Fiber isn't absorbed into the body, so it passes out of the body, taking the bile with it. Beans also help prevent blood sugar levels from rising too quickly after a meal, making beans a good food choice for people with diabetes or hypoglycemia. Combining beans with whole-grain rice gives you all the essential amino acid proteins.

A little-known and beneficial attribute of beans is that they contain the enzyme sulfite oxidase, which can detoxify sulfites. Sulfites are a common preservative used in many foods today. Many people are sensitive to sulfites. Sulfites in foods can cause some people to gain weight, and have headaches and rapid heartbeats. Eating one cup of black beans can give you 172% of the daily value of the trace mineral molybdenum, which is the key component of sulfite oxidase.

The *Journal of Agriculture and Food Chemistry* researched beans and found that they are as rich in anthocyanins, an anti-oxidant compound, as cranberries, oranges, and grapes. In fact, black beans had about 10 times the amount found in oranges. The darker the bean, the higher the anti-oxidant properties were. Gram for gram, black beans had the highest levels of anti-oxidants. They descended in order of black, red, brown, yellow, and lastly white.

Vegetarian Protein Sources

Almonds (¼ c.) 12 grams
Amaranth (3½ oz.) 16 grams
Baked beans (8 oz.) 11.5 grams
Broccoli (3½ oz.) 3.1 grams
Brown rice (7 oz.) 4.4 grams
Buckwheat (3½ oz.) 12 grams
Bulgar (1 c. cooked) 6 grams
Cashews (¼ c.) 5 grams
Chickpeas/garbanzo beans (7 oz.) 16 grams
Cow's milk (½ pint) 9.2 grams
Egg (boiled) 7.5 grams
Hard cheese (1 oz.) 6.8 grams
Hemp nuts (also called seeds) (1 oz.) 11 grams
Lentils (4½ oz.) 9.1 grams
Mediterranean pine nuts (1 oz.) 10 grams
Muesli (2½ oz.) 7.7 grams
Nori seaweed (3½ oz. dried) 35 grams
Nutritional yeast (3½ oz.) 50 grams
Oatmeal (1 c.) 6 grams
Peanuts (1 oz.) 7.3 grams
Pine nuts (1 oz.) 6.8 grams
Porridge (6 oz.) 2.4 grams
Potatoes (7 oz.) 2.8 grams
Pumpkin seeds (raw) (1 oz.) 7 grams
Sesame seeds (3½ oz.) 19 grams
Spinach (fresh) (1 c.) 1 gram
Spirulina (3½ oz.) 68 grams
Sunflower seeds (3½ oz.) 24 grams
Tofu (5 oz.) 10.3 grams
Walnuts (¼ c.) 25 grams
Whole-grain bread (2 slices) 7 grams

Raw and Living Foods

Raw foods are foods that have not been heated over 105–118 degrees. The enzymes in the food retain much higher nutrient levels in this form. It is all about enzymes. We need enzymes for digestion and nutrient absorption. Live enzymes in foods help foods to be digested more efficiently and completely. The key to health is a clean and nutrient-rich body.

Raw and living foods are the best form of foods for optimum health and wellness. These foods will feed the body on a deep cellular level without stressing the body as much as cooked food will. Cooked foods are dead. They don't supply any live enzymes, so your body has to work much harder, by supplying more of its own enzyme store, in order to digest them. Having to pull enzymes from the enzyme storage and working harder to supply them and use them to digest the "enzyme-empty" food is more work for the body (versus simply eating foods that supply their own enzymes readily for digestion).

Raw and living foods have more nutrients available for the body in digestion. Raw foods are also highly alkalizing. The body's pH should ideally be around 7.2 to 7.3. Most people with chronic or acute diseases usually have overly acidic bodies. Eating foods that are highly alkalizing can help the body maintain a healthier pH balance. What kinds of foods are in a raw and living food diet? Uncooked (not heated over 105 degrees) and unprocessed fruits, vegetables, nuts, seeds, and grains make up this diet. Fruit is such a pure form of food that it digests quickly compared to other foods, so it is best to eat fruit by itself and at least 15 to 30 minutes before eating other types of foods. A good number of the recipes in this book are raw and living food recipes.

Many people have started eating raw foods in order to heal their bodies or to just be healthier. Some clients who have come to work with me had adopted this diet on a 100-percent basis, and they were feeling sick and weak after being on the 100% raw food diet for about a year or two. If eating raw is taken to extremes, it can create an imbalance in the body and cause some stress on the thyroid, spleen, and/or pancreas. A diet varied with the amount of raw food eaten, eating with the seasons, and eating for your blood type can bring more balance to the body. Eating lighter raw foods in the warmer months and adding some warmer foods to the diet in the colder months can be more supportive to certain people and to certain parts of the body. For instance, the thyroid can be supported better when cruciferous vegetables like broccoli and cauliflower are lightly steamed instead of eaten raw. This is because these foods, as well as a few others, like yams, canola, and soy, contain natural chemicals called goitrogens that can interfere with thyroid hormone synthesis. Lightly steaming or cooking the vegetables will deactivate these chemicals. Adding foods like cooked whole-grain rice to the diet can work as a tonic for the spleen and/or pancreas.

A diet with a ratio of about 80 percent raw to 20 percent cooked food will work for most people, most of the year. Enjoy your raw foods, but remember to listen to your own body and create balance in your health, your diet, and your life.

Sugar: Watch Out for It!

Sugar consumption is out of control. Sugar is an ingredient that is in almost all processed foods, fast foods, and dairy products. I even see it added to dried fruits, trail mixes, and granolas in healthy grocery stores. According to the US government, the average American consumes on average ½ cup caloric sweeteners per day, or 152 pounds per year.[107] Sugar has the reputation of being "white poison" because of the harmful effects it has on the body's health. Although fat has been made out to be the cause of many diseases or problems, sugar is one of the most harmful ingredients in our diet.

Sugar can be hiding in many products you would not normally think. When food companies started making low-fat products, many added additional sugar to help the food taste more appealing. Studies conducted by the *American Journal of Clinical Nutrition* found that diabetes and obesity are directly linked to eating refined sugar and high-fructose corn syrup, the cheapest form of sugar and the choice of many food manufacturing companies.[108,109,110]

Along with diabetes and obesity, sugar intake can contribute to hypoglycemia, cardiovascular disease, kidney disease, high blood pressure, tooth decay, systemic infections, memory disorders, allergies, upset hormonal imbalances, and auto-immune and immune deficiency disorders. It supports the growth of cancer cells. The list of health problems goes on to include acne, adrenal gland exhaustion, allergies, anxiety, bloating, bone loss, eczema, cataracts, candidiasis, insomnia, ulcers, psoriasis, over-acidity, gout, gallstones, fatigue, menstrual difficulties, indigestion, high triglyceride levels, and more. These are all good reasons to limit the intake of sugar in one's diet.

Digestion breaks down the food we eat into glucose, and then the glucose is able to enter the blood stream. Through the blood stream, the glucose can enter the cells and be used for fuel, or stored in the liver or muscles for future use. Glucose is what powers every cell in the body. When glucose gets into the blood stream too quickly, blood sugar spikes and it puts pressure on the pancreas to make more insulin in order to regulate blood sugar levels. Insulin is a hormone the body makes in order to help maintain healthy glucose percentage levels in the blood. White refined sugar, high-fructose corn syrup, and fructose are very hard on the body and the digestive system. These sugars are read by the body as empty sugar. When the body consumes nutrient-empty sugar, the body has to pull stored nutrients out of the body in order to process the nutrient-empty sugar. This depletes the body of stored nutrients and can result in extreme cravings by the body for nutrients.

The body will only crave what it needs. Feeding the body empty calories of white refined sugars or carbohydrates can result in hunger pangs. Many people today who are walking around with extreme obesity or weight problems are actually walking around starving to death. Their bodies are not getting the nutrients they need. They may feel like they are so hungry and as a result eat more of the same, nutrient-empty food, which will overwork the pancreas and can result in the body having a tougher and tougher time creating the insulin to help make normal, healthy glucose levels. The constant roller coaster of blood sugar spiking can wear out the pancreas and therefore create less or no insulin at all. Also, an excess of glucose in the system can result in the storage of the excess glucose in the liver as glycogen. When the liver can't hold any more, it will return it to the blood stream as fatty acids. This can create insulin resistance, which can lead to diabetes. A diet of too much "empty sugars" on a continual basis can result in many diseases and obesity.

Sugar can affect health in negative ways. British psychiatric researcher Malcolm Peet conducted a study showing a diet high in sugar and its strong link to depression and schizophrenia by suppressing a key growth hormone in the brain called BDNF.[111] This hormone plays a vital role in memory function. It can be easy to get addicted to the short-lived sugar rush and energy-high feeling that eating sugary foods can create.

Since we are looking at the harmful effects of sugar on the body and brain, Dr. Francis Stern states, "A characteristic of sugar 'binges' is the taste for sweets for some reason leads to a craving for more of the same, just the way other drugs create cravings."[112] FDA Consumer reported in February 1988, "Drugs upset the body's homeostasis (balance) mechanism so completely that, in a struggle to get back to normal, the addict can only take another dose of the same drug. Heroin, cigarettes, coffee, sugar—it's the same kind of addiction."[113]

Sugar is like an addictive drug. Sugar can give the body an artificial energy surge, and the body can begin to crave that energy. Stimulants like caffeine or alcohol can cause sugar cravings. Today, large amounts of sugar are added to almost all packaged foods, including canned foods, jams, jellies, dry cereals, baked goods, breading, and dairy products. Read ingredient lists or simply to make your own food so that you know exactly what is in the food you are eating.

Sugar is a hidden ingredient in many foods today. In addition to the obvious reason—that it makes the food taste sweeter—added sugar also helps processed foods because it helps reduce shrinkage, keeps them smoother, and helps keep them from drying out. Here are just a few examples of foods in which you will find added sugar: seafood breading, canned salmon, hamburgers in restaurants, processed lunch meats, bouillon cubes, dry-roasted nuts, peanut butter, canned tomatoes, and canned vegetables.

According to Frances Sheridan Goulart, Glenn Craig, director of public information for Nabisco, Inc., admits that, although they aren't a dessert, even Nabisco Ritz Crackers contain 6% sweetening in the form of sucrose because "sugar is unmatched when it comes to making products tender and appetizing," according to the International Sugar Research Foundation (ISRF).[114]

It is very important to eat whole, unrefined foods that contain no or little white refined, processed sugar, high-fructose corn syrup, fructose, agave nectar, dextrose, glucose, fructose, maltose, barley malt, and sorbitol. Sugars are not all created equally, and some are far worse than others.

Here are a few types of sweeteners that are alternatives to white refined sugar. Some are good, and some aren't so good. Become sugar savvy!

Agave syrup is frequently used in many vegan and raw foods, because it is not taken from an animal. Agave is actually more calories than table sugar (20 to 16 per teaspoon). Agave is 90% fructose and is actually more fructose than what is used in high-fructose corn sweetener. Agave is commonly called "fructose sweetener." It is actually marketed as "diabetic friendly" because it doesn't have as much glucose in it as other sweeteners, but some studies suggest that large amounts of fructose can "promote insulin resistance (and thus increase diabetes risk, boost triglycerides (fats in the blood), lower HDL ('good') cholesterol, and have other harmful effects on the heart, and possibly the liver, too."[115] You may think, "But fructose is in fruit." Whole fruit contains added nutrients, fiber, and natural electrolytes, and affects the body in a different way than the refined agave syrup. In fact, agave syrup is made very much like high-fructose corn syrup, and a recent study showed it as having "minimal anti-oxidant activity." Agave is "just another form of processed (and concentrated) sugar," according to Berkeley Wellness Alerts.[116]

Blackstrap molasses is the residue of beet juice or sugar cane after the sugar crystals are removed. The molasses has minerals, including iron, calcium, and magnesium, even though it is still about 65% sucrose. Buy organic varieties.

Coconut sugar is made from boiling down the nectar of the tropical coconut palm sugar blossoms. This sugar has a naturally low glycemic index. This sugar has been used in the East Asian culture for herbal medicine and food preparation. The glycemic index is about 35. It is high in potassium, magnesium, zinc, iron, and B vitamins. Buy this sugar as organic, unprocessed, unbleached, and unfiltered with no preservatives.

Date sugar is derived from dried dates. This type of sugar has some fiber and is rich with minerals, since it is essentially dried fruit. It is a nice alternative to other sugars.

Honey is a natural sweetener that is anti-fungal, is antibacterial, can be used as a natural antiseptic, is a natural remedy for many ailments, and can boost energy. Honey contains a variety of nutrients and minerals, as well as some enzymes. It is known to help the facilitation of muscle recuperation and glycogen restoration after a workout. Honey is unique and can be substituted for sugar in recipes. *Weekly World News* listed arthritis, hair loss, bladder infections, upset stomach, indigestion, influenza, longevity, heart disease, colds, and cholesterol as some of the afflictions that could be cured by honey and cinnamon.[117] Always buy raw, unrefined honey, because it will have all of the live enzymes and nutritional properties still intact.

According to Ann Louise Gittleman, PhD, CNS:

> Never give an infant under eighteen months of age honey or products made with honey. This sweetener sometimes contains trace amounts of botulinum spores, which are easily denatured by the mature digestive tract of an adult but can be harmful or even fatal to an infant, whose digestive tract is just developing.[118]

Maple syrup is a natural sugar derived from maple tree sap that contains minerals including potassium and calcium.

Sucanat is dehydrated cane juice. This is an easy alternative to white refined sugar and is a small step in the direction of a healthier alternative to white refined sugar. Sucanat has some nutrients. It is made from taking the crystals from sugar cane juice that has had the water removed.

Stevia Rebaudiana Bertoni (known as ***stevia***) is a member of the aster family. Stevia is a sweet plant from South America. The stevia plant has been used commonly in Paraguay to treat diabetes and by indigenous populations for the control of fertility. You might want to keep this in mind if you are using stevia and you are young and trying to get pregnant. With regard to the control of fertility, Tufts University says that "some researchers have expressed concern that stevia might have an antifertility effect in men or women. However, evidence from most (though not all) animal studies suggests that this is not a concern at normal doses."[119] (The article does not say what the "normal" amount of stevia would be, but does include a section on dosage. The WebMed website says to simply follow the recommended dosage on the container.)

Japanese food manufacturers developed this sweetener in the 1970s for use in their products as a zero-calorie sugar. The Japanese have done extensive research on stevia and found it to be extremely safe. The less-refined varieties of stevia are the best in terms of health benefits. (Less-refined foods of any type are healthier than refined ones, because they are in a more natural, whole-food form.) Stevia is sold as a powder to be added to foods "as needed for appropriate sweetening effects."[120] As far as safety is concerned, Tufts University Medical Center reports: "Reassurance also comes from the study that found no effect with a dose of 15 mg/kg per day."[121]

Stevia comes in powder and liquid. I like the liquid form best. I think it has a better flavor. The powder form can be a bit bitter. I have been using this sweetener for years and absolutely love it in the liquid form. Make sure to read the ingredient label. Companies use different ingredients to preserve it or make it packagable. One company, for example, uses grapefruit seed extract. Grapefruit seed extract can interact very badly with some medications. Be aware of this and read all of the ingredients carefully, before using.

The WebMD website includes this information for drug interactions:

- Lithium interacts with STEVIA.
- Stevia might have an effect like a water pill or "diuretic." Taking stevia might decrease how well the body gets rid of lithium. This could increase how much lithium is in the body and result in serious side effects. Talk with your healthcare provider before using this product if you are taking lithium. Your lithium dose might need to be changed.
- Medications for diabetes (Antidiabetes drugs) interacts with STEVIA.
- Stevia might decrease blood sugar in people with type 2 diabetes. Diabetes medications are also used to lower blood sugar. Taking stevia along with diabetes medications might cause your blood sugar to go too low. Monitor your blood sugar closely. The dose of your diabetes medication might need to be changed. Some medications used for diabetes include glimepiride (Amaryl), glyburide (DiaBeta, Glynase PresTab, Micronase), insulin, pioglitazone (Actos), rosiglitazone (Avandia), chlorpropamide (Diabinese), glipizide (Glucotrol), tolbutamide (Orinase), and others.
- Medications for high blood pressure (Antihypertensive drugs) interact with STEVIA.

  Stevia might decrease blood pressure in some people. Taking stevia along with medications used for lowering high blood pressure might cause your blood pressure to go too low. However, it's not known if this is a big concern. Do not take too much stevia if you are taking medications for high blood pressure. Some medications for high blood pressure include captopril (Capoten), enalapril (Vasotec), losartan (Cozaar), valsartan (Diovan), diltiazem (Cardizem), Amlodipine (Norvasc), hydrochlorothiazide (HydroDIURIL), furosemide (Lasix), and many others.[122]

From what I gather from all of this information, this plant can help people who are trying to lower their blood pressure and/or blood sugar levels.

If you have any concerns, talk to your physician.

Xylitol is a sugar alcohol naturally found in fruits and vegetables that is usually made from birch tree bark and other hard wood trees. Xylitol was discovered by German scientist Emil Fisher in 1891. When Finland had severe sugar shortages during World War II, they started using it commercially. Finnish dentists noticed that schoolchildren had unusually strong teeth, free of cavities after the war. This discovery led the Finnish government to be the first to officially endorse the use of xylitol as a sweetener. By the 1960s, Germany, Switzerland, Japan, and the Soviet Union were using xylitol as their preferred sweetener for diabetics as well as an energy source for infusion therapy patients with impaired glucose intolerance and insulin resistance. Xylitol has a glycemic index of 7. Finnish scientists published over 200 medical studies of xylitol's effects between 1971 and 1999. Xylitol is considered a 5 carbon sugar. This means that it has antimicrobial effects of preventing the growth of bacteria. Xylitol is also alkaline-enhancing. Xylitol can replace sugar in recipes in an equal substitution. Xylitol tastes and looks just like sugar, and has no bitter aftertaste.

The only side effect that has been reported for xylitol is that, when consumed in large doses (over 30 or 40 grams at one time), it can cause gas and diarrhea. Drug interactions have not been found. Xylitol and stevia are both preferred sweeteners for diabetic diets. Many studies have been done on xylitol, and it has been shown to help prevent cavities, repair dental enamel, regulate blood sugar for those with type 2 diabetes, strengthen bones, decrease age-related bone loss, inhibit serious systematic yeast problems, inhibit the growth of bacteria that cause middle-ear infections in young children, inhibit the growth of streptococcus pneumonia, and alleviate dry mouth. Xylitol has 40% less calories and 75% fewer carbohydrates than sugar. Xylitol is slowly absorbed and metabolized, which results in negligible changes in insulin. Studies have shown that consumption of xylitol can reduce sugar cravings, reduce insulin levels, and alkalize your body. It was approved by the FDA in 1963.[123]

I recommend avoiding fake sugars and/or sugar substitutes altogether. Chemically derived sweeteners can have a harmful effect on health in many ways. Artificial sweeteners are never a healthy sugar alternative. All artificial, chemical sweeteners are toxic and can indirectly lead to weight gain, the very reason many people consume them.

They should be avoided. In fact, given a choice between high-fructose corn syrup and artificial sweeteners, high-fructose corn syrup is recommended by far (though it's essentially asking if you should consume poison or worse poison).[124]

Try to stay with real, whole, unrefined, or unprocessed sugars as much as possible. Read ingredient labels carefully, and check for any sugar or sugar substitute. Be knowledgeable about what you are eating.

"One farmer said to me 'Your body cannot live on vegetarian food solely, for it furnishes nothing to make the bones with;' and so he religiously devotes a part of his day to supplying himself with raw material of bones; walking all the while he talks behind his oxen, which, with vegetable made bones, jerk him and his lumbering plow along in spite of every obstacle."

~ Henry David Thoreau

Sulfites

Sulfites are preservatives that are added to many foods, drinks, and medicines. In fact, they have been used for centuries as a preservative because they preserve the color and flavor by inhibiting the growth of bacteria. Symptoms of sulfite allergy include weight gain, or the inability to lose weight, and respiratory types of problems. Many people who have been struggling with weight find that, after cutting out sulfites, they can lose weight much more easily and can then keep it off.

The most reliable way to test for sulfite allergy would be to go on a totally non-sulfite diet for several weeks. Because sulfites are hidden in many foods, you may have to eat nothing but whole, organic, non-sulfite or sulfate-agent-containing foods (in the forms of sodium sulfite, sodium bisulfite, sodium metabisulfite, metabisulfite, potassium bisulfate, and potassium metabisulfites) for three weeks. If all of your symptoms disappear, then you may be allergic to sulfites or another additive in the foods that you have cut out of your diet. Some doctors may want to give you a pill containing sulfites to see if the symptoms reoccur, just to confirm the allergy. (This should be done under close supervision.)

If you are allergic to sulfites, then you can simply regulate your diet accordingly to try to avoid sulfites. The USDA requires any food containing 10ppm or more of sulfites to be labeled, but since the labels on many foods change periodically, read the labels each time you buy processed food products. Look for sulfite, sodium bisulfite, sodium metabisulfite, potassium bisulfite, and potassium metabisulfite on labels.

Foods that commonly add sulfites to their ingredients are soups, canned vegetables, dried fruits, bakery items, pickles, potato chips, many condiments, trail mixes, shrimp, and guacamole. The FDA passed a law in 1986 banning the use of sulfites on raw fruits and vegetables. Vitamin C, quercetin, and bromelain are vitamins commonly used to aid in the treatment of sulfite allergies. Vitamin C and quercetin are immune system boosters. Bromelain will help your body use quercetin. Quercetin is also known for its ability to block the release of histamines, so it helps with any allergy symptoms.

You may find that you feel much better after you cut sulfites out of your diet. Removing the chemicals and preservatives out of the food you eat is a huge step toward getting healthier. Many of us grew up thinking that additives are "normal" to ingest, but, in my opinion, God did not make our bodies to assimilate chemicals and preservatives. Did God make a little baby and then say, "Please give this little baby chemicals and preservatives for nourishment"? Whole, real food that is grown, harvested, and stored in a safe and healthy way is what I believe we are meant to have as nourishment for our body.

Vitamin B

Although all nutrients and minerals are important for optimum health, there are a few nutrients that can be critical to health. One of those nutrients is Vitamin B.

Make certain that you are getting an adequate amount of all of the B vitamins. Thiamine (Vitamin B1), riboflavin (Vitamin B2), and niacin (Vitamin B3) are necessary for energy production.

"Vitamin B-5, or pantothenic acid, is a B vitamin that serves several important functions in the human body. This vitamin aids in the utilization of fats and proteins in food sources. Vitamin B-5 also aids in the conversion of carbohydrates into blood sugars, which your body uses for energy."[125] Foods that should contain Vitamin B5 are whole grains, legumes, eggs, nuts, fresh avocados, spinach, kale, broccoli, cauliflower, corn, and tomatoes.

Vitamin B6 helps your body process protein, as well as supports the nervous system and immune system. Vitamin B6 is in avocados, bananas, and eggs.

Biotin (Vitamin B7) helps the body produce hormones and aids in converting food into energy.

Folate (Vitamin B9) is also known as folic acid in its synthetic form. You want to purchase B vitamins with the folate whole-food form. Look for 5-methyltetrahydrofolate or 5-MTHF as the folate, and avoid supplements with folic acid. High intakes of folic acid have been associated with higher risks of cancer, as well as masking B12 deficiencies. Also, since B9 deficiencies can be so problematic,

> The Centers for Disease Control and Prevention recommends that vegetarian and non-vegetarian moms-to-be take 400 mcg folate supplement before and during pregnancy to ensure they are receiving an adequate amount to stave off potential birth defects. Folate can also be found in citrus fruits, peanuts and some mushrooms.[126]

Folate as well as Vitamin A is concentrated in green vegetables like romaine lettuce, spinach, turnip greens, mustard greens, parsley, collard greens, broccoli, cauliflower, beets, and lentils.

The B vitamin that I have found to be so vitally important for vegetarians in particular is Vitamin B12. Vitamin B12 is unique. "Microorganisms, primarily bacteria, are the only known organisms that manufacture B12. These bacteria often live in bodies of water and soil. Animals get B12 by eating food and soil contaminated with these microorganisms."[127] Vitamin B12 is almost exclusively found in animal sources. Plant food can have Vitamin B12 if it is taken from the earth, which contains some cobalt in it, and not cleaned, leaving the bacteria on it.

> Animals and plants require cobalt in order to synthesize/produce B12. (B12 is called cobalamin because of the cobalt atom in its center.) In reply to "where does the bacteria come from", one could maybe reply "from cobalt" but this isn't totally 100% correct. It comes from a combination of microorganisms and cobalt. B12 can sometimes be found on the surface of plants, and commercial B12 production is partly based on growing B12 on the surface of molasses. Animals need cobalt from the soil in order not to develop B12 deficiency.[128]

Eggs and dairy have some Vitamin B12. Vitamin B12 is so important for overall health. This is the main thing I tell anyone who is becoming a vegetarian, or who has been one and is not doing well. Have your blood checked by your doctor to make certain that you have the adequate requirements. I suggest having the doctor check all the B vitamins, including folate. According to the Physicians Committee for Responsible Medicine, the Vegan Society, and the Vegetarian Resource Group, vegans in particular should eat foods on a consistent basis that are fortified with Vitamin B12, or take a daily or weekly supplement. They also say that vegetarian and vegan adults over the age of 51 should consume foods or supplements that meet the RDA requirements, because they are more at risk for the deficiency. The recommended requirements from the RDA for vitamins are the minimum it takes for a person to survive. Remember that when taking vitamins, if you want to thrive. Also remember to only buy vitamins made from whole, organically grown foods. Foods that are fortified with B12 are usually some soy products and breakfast cereals.

To get the full benefit of a vegan diet, vegans should do one of the following:

- Eat fortified foods two or three times a day to get at least 3 micrograms (µg or mcg) of B12 a day, *or*
- Take one B12 supplement daily providing at least 10 micrograms, *or*
- Take a weekly B12 supplement providing at least 2,000 micrograms.

If you're relying on fortified foods, check labels carefully to make sure you are getting enough Vitamin B12. For example, if a fortified plant milk contains 1 microgram of Vitamin B12 per serving, then consuming three servings a day will provide adequate Vitamin B12. Others may find the use of Vitamin B12 supplements more convenient and economical. The less frequently you obtain Vitamin B12, the more you need to take, as Vitamin B12 is best absorbed in small amounts. The recommendations take full account of this. There is no harm in exceeding the recommended amounts or combining more than one option.

Symptoms of deficiency include

> loss of energy, tingling, numbness, reduced sensitivity to pain or pressure, blurred vision, abnormal gait, sore tongue, poor memory, confusion, hallucinations and personality changes. Often these symptoms develop gradually over several months to a year before being recognized as being due to B12 deficiency and they are usually reversible on administration of B12.[129]

When I read this list, I was really surprised. Lack of Vitamin B could have been one of the contributing factors to my vision problems. I have battled vision problems all of my life. I read this, too:

> According to optometrist Ben C. Lane of the Optical Society, there is a link between nearsightedness and chromium and calcium levels, which are lowered by sugar and protein consumption. Excessive intake of sugar and overcooked proteins exhaust the body's supplies of chromium and B vitamins. Fluid pressure in the eye, a contributing factor of nearsightedness, is regulated by the B vitamins.[130]

Make certain that you are getting adequate amounts of all of the B vitamins.

Vitamin D

Vitamin D is a prohormone that your body produces from cholesterol.

> Because it is a prohormone, vitamin D influences your entire body—receptors that respond to the vitamin have been found in almost every type of human cell, from your brain to your bones…it is also involved in multiple repair and maintenance functions, touches thousands of different genes, regulates your immune system, and much, much more…. Just one example of an important gene that vitamin D up-regulates is your ability to fight infections, as well as chronic inflammation. It produces over 200 anti microbial peptides.[131]

Vitamin D is essential for everyone, not just vegetarians. Studies show that about 85 percent of the US population is critically low in Vitamin D.[132] It may be the use of sunscreen, or the fact that most people work and stay indoors a good deal of the time, and therefore don't get enough direct sunlight without sunscreen. Get some sunshine! Get out in the sun every day for at least 20 minutes without sunscreen. The more skin is exposed, the more sunlight you can absorb. As we age, we need more Vitamin D. During the winter months, it may be harder or even impossible to get the amount of Vitamin D from the sun. Full-spectrum lighting indoors can really help with depression, mood, and health, but it is not a reliable source of Vitamin D.

Very few foods have good levels of Vitamin D, so a supplement is needed. Parsley, mushrooms exposed to ultraviolet light, fortified orange juice, and some milk actually do have some Vitamin D in them. Cod liver oil is the leading form of fish that contains Vitamin D, but this is not an acceptable way to ingest Vitamin D for vegetarians.

Vitamin D is an essential vitamin for health. Vitamin D deficiency has been linked to many diseases, including cancer. Check with your physician to make certain that the levels of Vitamin D in your blood are optimum.

Much controversy surrounds the Institute of Medicine's Food and

Nutrition Board's new claims (from limited studies) for the recommended daily allowance (RDA) of Vitamin D. Many doctors think it is recommending far too little.

> Heather Chappell of the Canadian Cancer Society (CCS) has stated that the organization will not lower their recommendations—which is currently 1,000 IUs per day, based on the vitamin D cancer research done by. Dr. Hearney and Lappe—because the IOM recommendations cover bone health only.... Bone health depends at least as much on vitamin D as on calcium.... And the CCS is still concerned about vitamin D deficiency and cancer.[133]
>
> So, how much vitamin D do studies suggest most U.S. residents need? Probably at least 1,000 IU per day, Holick and Heaney agree. Indeed, Heaney concludes in his October paper, if one accepts the 32 ng/ml value of 25-D as the necessary minimum for preventing bone loss in the United States, a minimum daily intake of some 2,600 IU of vitamin D per day would be needed to meet the needs of 97 percent of U.S. residents. That's well above the existing 400 to 600 IU intake recommended 8 years ago by the Institute of Medicine. That's why there's a move afoot to change vitamin D's recommended intake, says Heaney.[134]

According to Dr. Cannell, Dr. Lichtenfeld, spokesperson for the American Cancer Society, has indicated that Americans continue to wait for more randomized, control trials before addressing their Vitamin D deficiencies, even though a large number of epidemiology studies indicate that Vitamin D deficiency is a common finding in people of all age groups around the world. I had a friend whose back started to hurt so badly, he could barely stand it. Months later, after excruciating pain and unbelievable amounts of testing, they found that he was critically low in

Vitamin D! With some intense Vitamin D supplementation, he started to feel much better and is back to his healthy state of being. I get a good deal of sunlight every day and I live in Texas, so I thought I had an optimum level of Vitamin D in my body. I had my doctor test me, only to find out that I was on the low end of optimum. This was during summer, so I was so surprised! Keep an eye on your Vitamin D.

Water

Water is one key nutrient to our health and well-being. Our bodies are about 66–72% water. Blood uses the water to transport oxygen, nutrients, and antibodies to all parts of the body. Many illnesses are actually a result of dehydration. When we feel thirsty, we are already dehydrated. I always drink a glass of pure mineralized water as soon as I wake in the morning. When we wake up, our body is empty, so our body will absorb whatever we ingest like a sponge. Therefore, a glass of high-quality, mineral-rich water will be utilized more efficiently. I try not to drink it with meals, because it can water down the digestive enzyme juices, making it harder to digest the food. It is best between meals.

Fereydoon Batmanghelidj MD studied water while he was a prisoner in an Iranian jail. He treated and cured about 3,000 prisoners, using water and a little sea salt to treat what he called chronic intracellular dehydration. He found that most people are sick because of dehydration. He wrote many books on the subject after his release. The "water cure" that he prescribed is:

1. Sufficient water. Drink an ounce of water for every 2 pounds of body weight daily. This means that someone weighing 200 pounds should drink 100 ounces of water a day. This is in addition to any other beverages. Consume water first thing upon getting up in the morning and then drink it all day long on a continual basis every two hours.

2. Sea salt. Put 1/8 teaspoon of sea salt on the tongue with every 16 ounces of water. This is a key component in the "water cure." This is really important for people suffering from allergies or asthma; the salt acts like an antihistamine.

Almost all public water supplies have added chemicals to the water supply, including sodium fluoride and chlorine, both of which are poisons. Chlorine was the first poison developed for warfare. Chlorine also destroys the Vitamin E in the body and the good probiotics in the intestines. "Industrial chemist J.P. Bercz, PhD, showed in 1992 that chlorinated water alters and destroys unsaturated essential fatty acids (EFAs), [14] the building blocks of people's brains and central nervous systems."[135]

While showering or swimming in chlorinated water, the chlorine soaks into the skin cells. Our skin is our largest organ. That is why the patch is used to give medicines to people; they absorb directly into the skin and from there into the blood stream.

Research linking swimming in chlorinated pools to cancer and other medical conditions continues to make headlines. The latest such studies come from the Centre for Research in Environmental Epidemiology in Barcelona, Spain. They indicate, among other things, that swimming in a pool with chlorine may increase the risk of developing cancer and damage lungs.[136]

Sodium fluoride and fluorosilicic acid are common chemicals added to our municipal water supply. Studies were done for tooth decay prevention with calcium fluoride. The companies that had a by-product of sodium fluoride (that can be contaminated with lead and arsenic as well) are companies that make aluminum and fertilizers. Sodium fluoride is the fluoride that the government adds to the water supply. This is added on the pretext that it is good for our teeth and health, but dental studies were done using calcium fluoride, so this is a different type of fluoride from what is being added to the water supply. Fluoride has been used in Chinese medicine as a tranquilizer and also in many places as a rat poison.

According to Paul Connett, PhD, "Fluoride is a cumulative poison. On average, only 50% of the fluoride we ingest each day is excreted through the kidneys. The remainder accumulates in our bones, pineal gland, and other tissues. If the kidney is damaged, fluoride accumulation will increase, and with it, the likelihood of harm."[137] Fluoride affects the thyroid gland and all our enzymatic systems. Side effects from fluoride include weight problems, damage to our immune system, and other serious disorders. These chemically derived fluorides are completely different from naturally occurring fluoride.

Fluoride affects different people and ages differently. According to Connett:

> The level of fluoride put into water (1 ppm) is up to 200 times higher than normally found in mothers' milk (0.005–0.01 ppm) (Ekstrand 1981; Institute of Medicine 1997). There are no benefits, only risks, for infants ingesting this heightened level of

> fluoride at such an early age (this is an age where susceptibility to environmental toxins is particularly high).[138]

Sweden, Denmark, Holland, Germany, Belgium, Norway, and France do not put fluoride in their water. Some of these countries have made it illegal to add to the water supply.

Huge numbers of Safe Drinking Water Act violations are reported each year by water treatment facilities. Many areas have old, dirty water pipes, and even some really old lead pipes, transporting the water. *New Scientist* reported that a comprehensive survey of US drinking water showed that it contained an array of hormonally active chemicals like MTBE (methyl-tert-butyl-ether), a chemical found in fuel and a potential human carcinogen in high doses, and atrazine, a US pesticide that was banned in the European Union. Atrazine has been linked to reproductive problems in lab animals and is also linked to both breast cancer and prostate cancer.

In 2010, *National Geographic* reported that drinking water in schools in 27 states was contaminated with toxic substances including lead.[139] In 2009, the Associated Press analyzed data from the EPA and found the public water for about 100 school districts contained lead, pesticides, and other toxins.[140] If it is being pumped to schools, then it is probably being pumped into homes and businesses as well. Because of the state of our municipal water supply, a good water filter can be a beneficial purchase. I recommend purchasing one for the whole house. When we shower, we can absorb as many toxins from the water as we can from drinking about eight glasses of water, so a shower or bath filter is recommended as well.

I want to water my vegetable and herb gardens with pure water, so I bought a filter that takes out the chlorine and some other contaminants. It screws right on to the garden hose. You can buy it in the RV/outdoor department at many stores for about $25 dollars, and it will last about three to six months.

The Reverse Osmosis is a really good water filter system, but it takes everything out, even the good minerals you need in the water. It also makes the water very acidic. When drinking water, the body will pull minerals from the body in order to process the water if the water is void of minerals. Real, natural spring, well, or fresh water sources contain minerals and nutrients. When drinking purified bottled water, you can add some minerals (like a pinch of sea salt) to the water. When you do this your body won't need to pull minerals from your body in order to process the water.

There are different types of sea salt with different mineral content. Try a few different ones and see which ones you like the best. Celtic sea salt is supposed to be high in minerals. I like to use Bolivian Rose salt as well. Try to buy a solar dried salt or a mined salt. Mined salt may be cleaner and more nutrient-dense, because it is from oceans that were less polluted and a more nutrient-dense time. Also, put your water in glass containers. Some plastics can leach into the water.

The potentially hazardous chemical BPA is part of many plastic containers. BPA-containing plastic can leach into the water for various reasons, but one way is when the water-filled plastic container is left sitting in a hot car; the plastic gets hot and can literally leach the plastic into the water. Plastic can have many negative effects on the body. If you buy plastic, buy plastics marked with #2, #4, or #5 on the bottom. These are supposed to be safer. A stainless-steel bottle is another good option. Do not get aluminum.

Bottled water comes in a variety of choices. The EPA standards of the Clean Water Act do not apply to bottled water; there is very little regulation on bottled water, which is why I recommend having your own filter. According to the Natural Resources Defense Council, the bottled waters with a higher pH balance and more nutrients were Fiji, Evian, San Pellegrino, Volvic, Trinity Springs, and Perrier.[141] The reverse osmosis purified water by Coca Cola, Dasani, has magnesium (Epsom salts) added to it.[142]

What about "vitamin waters"? Many vitamin waters contain all kinds of ingredients, like high-fructose corn syrup, artificial color, preservatives, and even caffeine. Make certain to always read ingredient lists before you buy anything. Packaging can be very misleading.

You can also hydrate with good, high-quality fruits and vegetables that are high in natural water content, like cucumber, watermelon, celery, and carrots. They contain pure water that is rich with vitamins and minerals. Watermelon is 90% pure, clean water. When you have these real, whole fruits and vegetables as juices, you are getting natural electrolytes as well as hydrating fluids. Coconut water is a good choice for a hydrating drink.

One last note about water: Masaru Emoto was born in Japan. He became known for his studies of water and its ability to change when "words of intent" (negative or positive) were applied to water in various forms. His work is fascinating and shows that the environment of water directly affects its molecular structure. Mr. Emoto's book, *Messages of Water,* contains photographs showing the molecular structure of the water when he started and after he had applied words to the containers of water. His playing music affected the molecular structure of water as well. The water crystal experiments consisted of exposing water to various words, pictures, or music, and then freezing and photographing the molecular structure of the crystals with microscopic photography. Mr. Emoto claims there are "many differences in the crystalline structure of the water,"[143] depending on the source of the water. The waters were taken from various places all over the world. A water sample taken from a pristine mountain showed a geometric shape when it was frozen. When polluted water was studied, the water showed very different water molecules.

One of his first experiments with photographing water molecular structure was fascinating. He put water from the same exact source in identical plastic jugs and left them overnight with labels of words or sayings on them. The molecular structure of the water in the jugs with negative sayings changed and looked like pus. On the other hand, the molecular structure of the water in the jugs with positive words attached—words like love and gratitude—looked absolutely beautiful, like snowflakes. The comparison was really startling. You can go to his website (www.masaru-emoto.net/english/e_ome_home.html) and see some of the pictures. It is definitely something to think about.

Thinking about the words affecting the water in the jugs can cause a person to think about the effect of negative self-talk. What does that do to the water in our body or the water around us in our life? What does that mean? Food for thought? Water for thought?

Infused Water: A Nice Alternative to Sodas

Water is so crucial to our health, but sometimes we just want something with a little more taste to it. Infusing water can be easy, inexpensive, nutritious, and delicious.

When infusing water, make sure the fruits are cleaned completely with food-grade hydrogen peroxide, food-grade vinegar, or a really good vegetable wash—whether the fruit is organic or not. (Be cautious when using fruit slices from restaurants or bars. Studies and tests done on fruits and vegetables that are added to drinks in many of these establishments have tested high in bacteria and E. coli.)

Mint is wonderful for fresh, infused water. It invigorates the mind, refreshes the senses, has antiseptic qualities, aids in digestion, helps with the function of the liver, and can help with fresh breath. There are quite a few different types of mint, and each has a wonderful, fresh quality. Mint is extremely easy to grow in a pot or garden, so you can have mint very inexpensively and with very little work year-round. You can put mint in ice cube trays with some purified water to keep frozen and handy. These are nice for adding to teas, cool water drinks, cold soups, or sauces in the hot summer months. (I give them to my dog, and I think it really helps her have better dog breath!)

Orange, lemon, lime, and grapefruit slices all add a little zing to water as well as a bit of Vitamin C. Lemon balm and other herbs that you may be particularly fond of are all healthful and fun to drink or use in recipes that call for water.

Infused water has very few calories and is a wonderfully healthy and fun way to enhance enjoyable refreshing water.

Zinc

Zinc is one of the most important minerals used by the body. It helps with the production of about 100 enzymes and contributes to building up the immune system.

It is required for protein and DNA synthesis, insulin activity, and liver function.

Zinc is not really stored in our body, so we need a regular supply. Zinc is found in our entire body. Men need more zinc than women (the recommended amount for men is one-third higher than for women) because the prostrate gland and semen are highly concentrated with zinc. Sexually active men need a good supply of zinc consistently.

A zinc deficiency may appear as skin problems, impairment of taste, a poor immune system, hair loss, diarrhea, fatigue, wounds not healing properly, or a poor or slow growth rate for infants. One reason for supplementation is that phytic acid and dietary fiber in certain foods can inhibit the absorption of zinc. So even if you are eating zinc-rich foods, the phytic acid may keep it from being absorbed by the body. Also, if the body has high levels of cadmium, then it will compete with the zinc to be absorbed. We can get cadmium in various ways, one being second-hand cigarette smoke. Other chemicals added to processed foods will also impair the absorption of zinc by the body.

Good sources of zinc are lentils, peas (chickpeas are good), seeds (sesame tahini paste is good, and so are pumpkin seeds), whole-grain cereals or breads, beans, cheddar cheese, yogurt, and wheat germ. Some fair sources are peanut butter, peas, figs, Brazil nuts, oranges, and almonds.

Make sure any supplements you take are high-quality, whole-food supplements.

Part II
Recipes

A Few Notes About Cooking and Food Preparation

Use a recipe book as a guidebook. Everyone's kitchen is different. Stoves are different and will cook at slightly different temperatures. The recipe creator's oven may cook faster or slower than yours. Keep this in mind whenever you are baking something. Different climates can affect the food and how it works in different recipes.

The quality of the ingredients is paramount to the quality of the dish and the taste of the food. A recipe tastes really satisfying if it has sweet, salty, sour or bitter, savory, and spicy in it. If a recipe is not quite right, see if you can add one of these to it to make it taste more delicious. Using all of these in a recipe will give it balance. Once you feel comfortable with the knowledge of what the healthier foods to eat are, start experimenting with your recipes.

One thing I do when I am "cooking" food is to try to save half of the raw vegetables and add them to the finished, cooked food as an additional way of adding some living enzymes into the dish. If I'm using a jarred tomato sauce, for example, I add some freshly chopped tomatoes, onions, and/or herbs to the final product for a fresher food with some living enzymes that can benefit my health. Look at the recipes that you are creating and see where you can do this. It makes dishes taste so much fresher and more alive!

Don't waste the tops, tips, and leftovers of the vegetables used in recipes. Use them to make a vegetable broth that you can use later. Simply place the leftover ends and tips in a pot of water, and bring to a boil. Add a little kombu seaweed if you have any. After it comes to a boil, reduce the heat and simmer 10 minutes or more. Remove from heat and strain off the broth. Put the broth in containers like ice cube trays and freeze them. This way you can pop out a couple cubes whenever you need some extra flavor in a dish.

Fruits and Vegetables

When buying fruit, look for firm, smooth, colorful fruit. The antioxidants are in the color; the more colorful the fruit, the higher the antioxidant content. Store fruit in a cool, shady place or the refrigerator until you want to eat it. Wash it right before you eat it. Place purified water in a bowl large enough for the fruit with a good fruit and vegetable rinse or some food-grade hydrogen peroxide. Apple cider vinegar is also a good fruit and vegetable cleaner. Use about a tablespoon for each gallon of water or one-quarter cup for a sink full of water. Soak fruit for about 15 minutes. Remove and dry. I clean all fruits and vegetables whether I peel them or not. The knife pulls all germs through the fruit when cutting. The fruit has been handled by pickers, in boxes, trucked, unpacked, and placed on shelves; it is always good to remove any dirt, germs, or debris from our food.

If you have fresh food from your garden that has been grown totally organically in organic soil, has already rinsed by fresh rain, and has not been handled by anyone else, and you know absolutely that this food is clean, it may be better to *not* rinse and clean it with a germ-killing rinse, because it will have some natural Vitamin B12 on it from the earth.

Grains, Roots, and Herbs

Grains should be kept dry, cool, and in a sealed container.

When ready to use, rinse grains. (I use a really fine mesh colander.) Grains have been milled, stored, and shipped. Bugs, mice, rats, and snakes can be found in storage units and silos.

Rinsing rice and other whole grains before you cook them helps remove a good portion of the starch. If you soak them for a few hours or overnight, they can sprout, and you will get a nutrient-activated grain that is more digestible.

Store garlic and ginger root in a dry, cool, and dark place.

Store oils and nuts in the refrigerator. Because they can become rancid, storing them in the refrigerator will keep them fresher longer.

Fresh herbs will stay alive and fresher longer when put in a vase like flowers with some water (and they look really nice as well!). You can keep them out on a table. I love to put fresh mint in a vase of water and snip off little bits of it periodically for mint-infused water or tea. Add a fresh flower and it is a beautiful arrangement for the kitchen.

Play and have some fun with your food!

Beverages

Juices and Juicing

When we juice foods, we get the nutrient density without the fiber. This way it is easier for the body to absorb; the body really doesn't have to work hard to get the benefits. This is extremely beneficial for someone who needs intense nutrition and isn't able to consume whole food or hardly any food. We can get intense nutrients with living enzymes to feed our cells on a deep cellular level when juicing. Fresh juice alkalizes us and flushes out the toxins in our cells. The highly anti-oxidant-rich nutrients are an amazing way to cleanse the body of toxins. A juice cleanse can be a great way to boost your energy, balance your blood sugar, brighten your skin, and rejuvenate your hormones. I love to juice green wheatgrass and barley grass, sunflower sprouts, and various other chlorophyll-rich foods. Nutrients start to disperse after about 20 minutes, so drink the freshly juiced juice immediately. "Vegetable juice is HIGHLY perishable so it's best to drink all of your juice immediately," according to Dr. Joseph Mercola.[144] When buying fresh juice, make sure the juice is made for you right then (not the night or morning before).

It is amazing how full you can feel after drinking a large glass of vegetable or fruit juice. I try to juice at least once a day. I usually have at least three carrots in my juice. When I am cutting vegetables, I save the pieces I don't use for my next juicing (the end of the celery, the rind of the watermelon, the base of the lettuce, the stalks of the broccoli, etc.). I juice almost all of the skins. The only skins I don't juice are melons like cantaloupe, because they are prone to mildew. Watermelon and citrus fruits are awfully powerful. You can juice them, but they are really strong-tasting. I have juiced whole lemons when I am juicing a good bunch of heavy greens. The lemons give your fresh juices with lots of greens a kick and take out some of the heavy green taste. I always make sure I have cleaned my fruits well, especially if I am juicing the skin.

Juicing can be an excellent way of fasting. You can get great nutrient density without all of the calories. This is also a good way to diet, without the intense hunger pangs. Just juice, juice, and juice for life!

Wheatgrass is a unique and beneficial food to juice. Dr. Yoshihide Hagiwara, president of the Hagiwara Institute of Health in Japan, advocates the use of grass as food and medicine. One reason is that grass is rich in chlorophyll. Chlorophyll is very similar to hemoglobin, a compound in blood that carries oxygen. Ann Wigmore wrote *The Wheatgrass Book*. Some of the benefits of drinking freshly juiced wheatgrass on a regular basis, according to Wigmore's book, are that it:

- Increases red blood cell count and lowers blood pressure.
- Cleanses the blood, organs, and gastrointestinal tract of debris.
- Stimulates metabolism and the body's enzyme systems by enriching the blood.
- Aids in reducing blood pressure by dilating the blood pathways throughout the body.
- Stimulates the thyroid gland, correcting obesity, indigestion, and a host of other complaints.
- Restores alkalinity to the blood. The juice's abundance of alkaline minerals helps reduce over-acidity in the blood.
- Can be used to relieve many internal pains and has been used successfully to treat peptic ulcers, ulcerative colitis, constipation, diarrhea, and other complaints of the gastrointestinal tract.
- Is a powerful detoxifier, and liver and blood protector. The enzymes and amino acids found in wheatgrass can protect us from carcinogens like no other food or medicine.
- Strengthens our cells, detoxifies the liver and bloodstream, and chemically neutralizes environmental pollutants.
- Neutralizes toxic substances like cadmium, nicotine, strontium, mercury, and polyvinyl chloride.
- Offers the benefits of a liquid oxygen transfusion since the juice contains liquid oxygen. Oxygen is vital to many body processes. It stimulates digestion (the oxidation of food), promotes clearer thinking (the brain utilizes 25% of the body's oxygen supply), and protects the blood against anaerobic bacteria. Cancer cells cannot exist in the presence of oxygen.[145]

Recent studies show that wheatgrass juice has a powerful ability to fight tumors without the usual toxicity of drugs that also inhibit cell-destroying agents. The many active compounds found in grass juice cleanse the blood, and neutralize and digest toxins in our cells. Dr.

Bernard Jensen, a renowned nutritionist, wrote *Health Magic Through Chlorophyll from Living Plant Life,* in which he mentions several cases in which his patient's red blood cell count doubled in a matter of days, just by soaking in a chlorophyll-rich bath. He says that blood builds more quickly when the person drinks the chlorophyll-rich fresh juices on a regular basis.[146]

There are some really good juicers on the market. A juicer is an investment, but it will give you really dense nutrients that are so beneficial to health. I think the hand-turn wheatgrass juicer is the best choice. It is less expensive and more reliable. Large juicers usually don't do grasses. Grass juicers don't handle large vegetables very well. You really need to have two different types of juicers: one for the grasses, and one for large fruits and vegetables. (Check the Resources for types of juicers.)

Juicing is great for everyone. For people who are trying to heal from various diseases, it can be especially powerful, with all of its nutrient-rich, anti-oxidant enzymes! For diabetics, the following foods have an insulin-type of action ("Insulin is a hormone secreted by your pancreas, and its function is to regulate blood glucose levels. Insulin works like a key to open the door of the cells so glucose—the fuel you get from food—can come inside and be converted into energy."[147]): asparagus, avocados, bitter melon, black pepper, Brussels sprouts, carrots, cinnamon, cucumbers, fennel, garlic, ginger, grapefruit, guava, parsnips, raw green vegetables, onions, leeks, sweet potatoes, tomatoes, winter squash, wheatgrass, sprouts, and yams. These are good choices for diabetics (or anyone, really). Just pick a few and vary them with the seasons as often as you can. At the Tree of Life, where I studied raw food and organic gardening, they did not put carrots in the juices for diabetics because of the higher sugar content of the vegetable; keep this in mind if you are a diabetic. Gabriel Cousens, MD, who wrote *There Is a Cure for Diabetes,* believes in and promotes juicing. In his book, he talks about juice feasting. What I found out about juicing is that when I am drinking these fresh, nutrient-dense juices, I never feel hungry or tired.

Protein Types and Juicing

For people with O blood types, which are known as protein types, Dr. Mercola said:

> If you are a protein type, juicing needs to be done cautiously. Celery, spinach, asparagus, string beans and cauliflower would be your best vegetables to juice. You can add some dark leafy greens like collards, kale, and dandelion greens but do so cautiously and pay careful attention to how you feel.
>
> You may also want to initially limit your serving size of juice to no more than 6 oz., and store it properly and drink smaller amounts throughout the day.
>
> Also, to make drinking vegetable juice compatible with protein type metabolism (which needs high amounts of fat), it is important to blend a source of raw fat into the juice. Raw cream, raw butter, raw eggs, avocado, coconut butter, or freshly ground flax seed are the sources of raw fat that we most recommend.
>
> In addition to adding a source of raw fat to your juice, you may also find that adding some, or even all, of the vegetable pulp into your juice helps to make drinking the juiced vegetables more satisfying.[148]

Interestingly, I had been adding about a tablespoon of pulp back into my juice, before reading this. I also add about a teaspoon of hemp oil, chia seeds, flax seed oil, or coconut oil to my smoothies and juices. I had been listening to my body and knew what it needed, even before I knew why. It is so important to get connected, really listen to your body, and find out what works best individually.

Greens are a powerhouse of nutrients. They have potassium, phosphorus, calcium, magnesium, iron, and zinc, along with vitamins A, C, E, and K. They have folic acid, chlorophyll, and micronutrients. Are you thinking, "Oh my goodness, greens for breakfast"? Yes! They are full of fiber. In traditional Asian medicine the color green is related to the liver, emotional stability, and creativity. Greens aid in purifying the blood, strengthening the immune system, and improving liver, gall bladder, and kidney function. The nutrients in greens can help fight depression, clear congestion, and improve circulation, which can help keep skin clear and blemish-free.

Celery is a natural electrolyte and is very hydrating. Carrots are a good blood regulator. They are beneficial to people with eye problems. Cucumbers are full of nutrients and natural electrolytes. Cucumbers are great for nourishing the skin. Watermelon is a great diuretic. Kale is known as the king of greens. Writing about kale and its benefits, Diane Dyer, MS, RD, says:

> The standouts are the high content of calcium, vitamin C, vitamin B6, folic acid, vitamin A (in the form of beta-carotene), vitamin K, potassium, manganese, copper, and even the plant form of omega-3 fatty acids (alpha-linolenic acid). In addition to the carotenoid beta-carotene, kale contains other very important carotenoid molecules called lutein and zeaxanthin (both necessary for eye health) and numerous others (probably too many to count, and maybe even yet identified).[149]

Just a note about sea salt and potassium: A person needs 1/8 teaspoon salt (3/4 gram) for every 8 ounces (250 cc) orange juice for the potassium to be used by the cells in the body, according to Jim Bolen in his paper "Histamine/Anti-histamine and the Dangers of Taking Anti-histamine."[160] Organic juice is loaded with potassium that our bodies cannot use without salt. Thus, when a person drinks orange juice and does not take enough salt, which is required for the potassium to go into the human cell, histamine is released to take care of the problem. When histamine is released, symptoms like hay fever, itching, nausea, vomiting, and sleep disorders can be some of the symptoms. But when potassium is properly absorbed, it aids the body with a natural antihistamine effect, thereby combating the above-mentioned histamine symptoms. Dr. Batmanghelidj, mentor to the above-mentioned Jim Bolen, explains this very clearly in his books.

In Dr. Batmanghelidj's book *ABC of Asthma, Allergies and Lupus,* he writes:

> It is a good policy to add some salt to orange juice to balance the actions of sodium and potassium in maintaining the required volume of water inside and outside the cells... In some cultures, salt is added to melon and other fruits to accentuate their

> sweetness. In effect, these fruits contain mostly potassium. By adding salt to them before eating, a balance between the intake of sodium and potassium results. The same should be done to other fruits.[151]

Some foods need to be lightly steamed before ingesting because they contain phytic acid, which acts like an anti-nutrient, so they may not be good choices for juicing. (The phytic acid will reduce the absorption of valuable minerals such as calcium, magnesium, and zinc.) Foods containing phytic acid are blackberries, broccoli, cauliflower, carrots, figs, and strawberries. The vegetables must be lightly steamed or cooked to help neutralize the phytic acid.[152]

The five goitrogenous chemicals in broccoli can disrupt the body's ability to use iodine. This can be a problem if someone has a thyroid deficiency or low iodine.[153]

Tomatoes are best when vine ripened. If tomatoes are green-picked and later ripened, they "can weaken the kidney–adrenal function."[154]

Spinach, beet greens, and chard are high in oxalic acid. These particular greens should be "taken in limited quantities by those with mineral deficiencies or loose stools because of the laxative effect and the calcium-depleting effect of their substantial oxalic acid content."[155] Oxalic acid binds with calcium. When it does this, if there isn't a good source of calcium consumed with the food, the body will pull it from the bones. When this occurs, it can be harmful to the kidneys. The oxalic acid can also affect the absorption of iron. Also, when eating spinach, have some Vitamin C–rich food with it to help the body absorb the iron in the spinach more efficiently.

I like to add a little coconut water, kefir, or kombucha to my drinks as an added benefit for my immune system. I don't have that listed in the recipes throughout the book, but you can add the probiotics or "fermented drinks" with the beneficial flora to support the immune system. I think it is really important to have it in the morning, when the body is empty and has the ability to absorb it more readily.

Raw recipe

BASIC GREEN DRINK

Ingredients:

1 c. fresh leafy greens
½ cucumber
juice of half a lemon
1 or 2 dates (non-sulphured), pitted and soaked in water for an hour
2 c. water

Directions:

1. Place all ingredients in a powerful blender and blend.

Notes:

1. Greens can be romaine lettuce, spinach, kale, beet greens, or a combination of any of these. Kale is an excellent choice. You may want to lightly blanch or steam the spinach to reduce the concentration of oxalic acid that it contains.
2. If you love lemon or citrus, add more lemon juice.
3. Drink this within 20 minutes of making.

Variation:

Substitute lime juice for lemon.

Raw recipe

INFUSED WATER

Ingredients:

4 c. high-quality water
1/8 c. fresh mint leaves, orange slices, or cucumber slices

Directions:

1. Combine all ingredients.
2. Let set for an hour or more.
3. Drain leaves or fruit out of the water, leaving only the water.

Notes:

1. This recipe is easy to double or triple.
2. This beverage is wonderful to serve at parties, at group meetings, after a workout, or to children as an alternative to sodas. Place a pretty slice or sprig of mint to the serving glass as a garnish.
3. Consume at room temperature or refrigerate for a cooler beverage.

Raw recipes

TASTY, HEALTHY JUICES!

Directions for all Juicing Recipes:

Juice ingredients and consume within 20 minutes for maximum nutritional benefit.

Recipe #1

Ingredients:

Wheatgrass or barley grass

A 2-ounce shot of this is rejuvenating.

Recipe #2

Ingredients:

Wheatgrass, sunflower sprouts, and pea sprouts

Juice wheatgrass and fresh sprouts as a regular morning juice for exceptional nutrition and health benefits.

Recipe #3

Ingredients:

Sunflower seed sprouts, mixed sprouts, cucumber, and celery

Recipe #4

Ingredients:

3 carrots, 2 or 3 cups whole kale or romaine lettuce, and 2 celery stalks

Recipe #5

Ingredients:

2 carrots, 1 cucumber, and 1 tomato

Recipe #6

Ingredients:

Peeled pineapple, peeled mango, peeled kiwi, apple without the seeds, and peeled orange

Recipe #7

Ingredients:

2 peeled kiwis, 2 celery stalks, a handful of berries of choice, 2 carrots, and 1 peeled orange

Notes:

1. Add a little (2 T.) fresh barley grass, ginger root, parsley, or cilantro to any of these juices for an extra nutrient kick!

2. If you don't like the heavy green taste, add lemon (I add a half of a lemon, including the skin) to the juice mixture to help cut that "green" taste. The lemon will add an extra bit of Vitamin C and is super-alkalizing.

Raw recipe

WARM LEMONADE

I drink this three or four times a week when I get up, before I have had anything else.

In nutrition school, I learned that drinking a cup of freshly squeezed lemon juice with warm water, first thing in the morning on a totally empty stomach, cleanses the organs and flushes out bacteria. It gives you a nice burst of Vitamin C and is alkalizing as well. Even though it may seem like a citrus fruit would be acidic, the body reads it as alkalizing. Sometimes I do lime or grapefruit juice, just for a change. It is really refreshing.

Ingredients:

½ lemon

1 c. water

Directions:

1. Juice lemon.
2. Warm up water (not hot) on a stovetop.
3. Combine lemon juice and water.

Note:

Drink within 20 minutes.

Variation:

For an extra treat, as your own version of "lemonade," if you don't have candida yeast problems or diabetes, add a teaspoon of honey. (The honey also has antibacterial properties.) If you have a problem with candida or diabetes, add a drop or two of liquid stevia to sweeten.

Raw recipe

WATERMELON DRINK

The heat of the summer is the perfect time to indulge in sweet, juicy, nutrient-rich watermelon. Watermelon is luscious and refreshing as a snack or as part of a fruit salad, dessert, or drink. One cup of watermelon has only 48 calories. However, it has high levels of nutrients, making it the perfect healthy treat. Watermelons are packed with Vitamin C, Vitamin A, vitamins B6 and B1, potassium, and magnesium. In addition, medical studies have shown that watermelon can help with inflammation conditions like asthma, atherosclerosis, diabetes, colon cancer, and arthritis. It is also high in the anti-oxidant lycopene, which has cancer-preventing properties and helps oxidize cholesterol.

Ingredients:

1 watermelon
a few limes, freshly juiced
pinch of whole sea salt

Directions:

1. Cut watermelon into chunks and remove seeds.
2. Place watermelon chunks in a blender.
3. Add a splash of fresh lime juice and a pinch of sea salt.

Notes:

1. Depending on the size of the watermelon, this can make a whole pitcher of drinks.
2. Store whatever is not consumed immediately in the refrigerator.

Variation:

Add some sparkling water and a spring of mint for a fresh cocktail.

Tea

Legend has it that tea was discovered by Chinese emperor Shen Nung in 2737 BC. His servant was boiling water under a tree and some leaves blew into the water. Shen Nung, a renowned herbalist, decided to try the infusion, and this resulted in what we now call tea. So, tea is hot water that is infused. Dried leaves or flowers are commonly packaged these days as tea.

Making tea is easy. Place 1 teaspoon of tea or one tea bag in a tea pot or tea cup, add a cup or two of hot water, and steep for two to five minutes. Drink it plain, or add a drop or two of stevia or honey for sweeter tea. You can also add a squeeze of fresh lemon juice or a spring of mint for added flavor.

Tulsi Tea

Tea is a great way to hydrate and get the benefit of various healing and soothing herbs. When I was working on our book, *Alive and Cooking,* with my friend and co-author Maryann De Leo, she came to stay with me for a week. She brought some tulsi tea with her. We drank a variety of tulsi teas all week long. They were absolutely delicious. I have found that I love the tulsi tea, a tea that has been used by the Ayurvedic practice for centuries and has been documented as far back as 5000 BC. In fact, this tea is at the heart of India's Ayurvedic holistic health practice. In India, the tulsi plant is sacred. It is known for promoting a healthier respiratory system and healthier vision, as well as reducing stress. Dr. Singh, author of *Tulsi—Mother Medicines of Nature,* said in his book that it is one of the best stress adaptogens. This means it can help you relax and stay calm, and can boost your system to handle stress better. Tulsi is supposed to balance the health of the digestive system, promote a healthy metabolism, support skeletal and joint support, help normalize cholesterol levels, boost stamina, help with mucus problems, and protect against free radicals.

Tulsi tea comes in a variety of flavors. I served one of my tulsi teas to a client one day and, about an hour after he left, he called me and asked, "What was that drink you gave me? I feel like Superman!" I told him that it was tulsi tea. He went right out and bought two or three different varieties. He now drinks it almost every day.

Raw recipe

GINGER TEA

One of my favorite teas that is great for the immune system, digestive system, and circulatory system is ginger tea. This can be especially good for anyone having digestive issues. You can buy ginger root at the grocery store, usually by the root vegetables or mushrooms. The skin should be smooth and tight, not wrinkly. The root should be firm. You can buy pieces of the root in all different sizes. Keep it in a cool, dry, dark place.

Ingredients:

1-inch-piece fresh ginger root
2 c. or more of hot water
stevia or raw honey to sweeten (optional)

Directions:

1. Grate or thinly slice ginger root.
2. Pour warm or hot water over it and steep about 5 minutes.
3. Strain.
4. Add a few drops stevia or honey, if using.

Raw recipe

TURMERIC "TEA"

Turmeric is a wonderful spice for restorative properties, including anti-inflammatory, anti-oxidant, and antimicrobial properties. It is a great blood purifier, and it helps hydrate dry skin. My daughter, Amanda, came home one day and said she had been adding ½ teaspoon or so to a cup of warm (not boiling) water and drinking it as a tea. It is really not an "official" tea, but that is what we call it. She made me some and I have been drinking it ever since!

In fact, what I do is I make this tea and drink it while I am letting my other tea steep, then I drink my other tea.

Milk Alternatives

Flavors and Sweeteners for Alternative Milks

For all of these milks, you can make them flavored if you wish. Here are a few ways to make them sweeter or more flavored:

1. Sweet Leaf brand stevia comes in flavors: orange, vanilla, toffee, and several others. They have no calories and are healthy. This is my sweetener of choice.

2. Add a dash or more of vanilla extract, maple extract, or almond extract.

3. Add a dash of cinnamon or a little grated orange zest for a bolder flavor. Cinnamon tastes good with orange, and you can do lemon or lime as well. With lemon or lime, you may want to add a tiny bit of maple syrup, honey, or a few more dates.

4. You can make many different flavors by adding any infused water.

5. Coconut water can be used to soak the cashews and added as the water for a wonderful coconut cream. Add a tiny bit of vanilla to this mixture.

Raw recipe

ALMOND MILK

I use this milk for many things, including as the liquid in my smoothies. I make my milk without sweetener and then add what I need to make it sweeter, depending on what I am using it for. I like to add a few drops of stevia most of the time. To flavor nut milks for drinking or to use on granola, I like to use the toffee stevia drops by Sweat Leaf. If I am using it for a recipe, I use plain stevia. My friend Maryann (with whom I co-authored the book *Alive and Cooking*) likes vanilla-flavored stevia. It is just a matter of personal opinion; find out what your favorite is!

Ingredients:

1 c. almonds, soaked in a bowl of water, refrigerator 12 to 18 hours and rinsed

3 c. water

Directions:

1. Blend soaked almonds with water until smooth.
2. Strain mixture through a sprout bag, cheesecloth, or strainer into a big bowl.

Notes:

1. This milk will last in the refrigerator for about three to five days. Shake well before using.
2. Save the almond pulp in a container and put in the refrigerator or freezer for later use. I use it to make my raw breads and crackers.
3. Almonds are soaked in water to remove the phytic acid.

Variations:

1. For a sweeter version, take a vanilla bean, split it, and scrape out the seeds. Add the seeds to the almond milk in the blender. Then add two or three dates, or another sweetener (like stevia), and blend until smooth.
2. Use a flavored stevia (like the ones by Sweet Leaf).
3. Substitute walnuts for almonds.

Raw recipe

CASHEW CREAM OR MILK

I started experimenting with different nut milks and found that I really like the creamy texture of cashews. You can make all kinds of wonderful recipes with this mixture as milk. I like to soak the nuts overnight in the refrigerator, but if you soak them a minimum of two hours, they will get soft enough to make a really nice milk when mixed in the blender. I add extra water to make it less creamy and milkier. This mixture is great with granola cereals. I try to keep a fresh mixture of this in my refrigerator at all times. I make it fresh about every three days. If you add some other flavors to it, it can make a nice cream for desserts and cereal toppings.

You can make any amount of this. This recipe makes a small amount (about ½ cup) to start, and you can double this recipe easily.

Ingredients:

1 c. cashews, preferably raw and organic
1½ c. water (for soaking the nuts at least two hours or overnight)
½ c. water (for adding to blender)

Directions:

1. Drain nuts after soaking in 1½ c. water.
2. Blend nuts and ½ c. water water in blender until smooth and creamy.
3. Add water to the desired consistency. (Add the amount of liquid as you go. You can make it thicker, like a cream, or you can make it thinner, like milk.)

Variations:

1. For a sweeter cream, add a date or two with the pit removed that has been soaked in just enough water to cover at least 30 minutes. Always add soaking water to the blender as well as dates.
2. For a sweet flavor, add Sweet Leaf brand stevia sweetener, which comes in many flavors. It has no calories and is healthy. This is my sweetener of choice. In this cream, I love the toffee flavor. Vanilla is also really good.
3. Add a dash of vanilla extract, maple extract, or almond extract.
4. Use coconut water to soak the cashews and add as the water for a wonderful coconut cream.
5. Add a tablespoon or more of fruit juice, like apple with a dash of cinnamon or orange juice (with a grated zest of the rind for a bolder flavor). Cinnamon tastes good with the orange flavor; you could do lemon or lime as well. With the lemon or lime, you may want to add a tiny bit of maple syrup, honey, or a few more dates.

Raw recipe

OAT MILK

This is very much like rice milk, only I use raw, uncooked oats. I use non-flavored stevia and omit vanilla if I am using the oat milk in a recipe.

Ingredients:

½ c. raw whole oats
1½ c. water
1 vanilla bean
stevia to taste
dash of sea salt

Directions:

1. Soak oats for 12 hours in 1 cup of the water called for in the ingredient list. This will help remove the phytic acid. Pour off any water when it is finished soaking.

2. Split vanilla bean and use a sharp knife to scrape out the inside of the bean. Put scrapings in a blender.
3. Combine all ingredients in a blender and blend well.
4. Strain through a nut milk bag or simply drink as a thicker, more fiber-filled version.

Variations:

1. Add more oats for a thicker milk.
2. Omit or use an alternative vanilla flavor for this milk, such as flavored stevia.
3. Add a handful or a few tablespoons of pine nuts or walnuts for a richer flavor.

Raw recipe

PINE NUT MILK

This is very much like rice milk, only I use pine nuts. You can use no sweetener or no flavored stevia, if you want to use this in a recipe. This is a thin nut milk, but you can add a few more nuts to make it thicker. Mediterranean pine nuts have more protein in them than any other nut. Pine nuts also have a unique ability to make you feel full and satisfied. They are great to have in the diet, if you need weight control. They can be expensive, but a little goes a long way.

Ingredients:

1 vanilla bean
½ c. raw pine nuts, soaked in water 12 to 18 hours and drained
1½ c. water
stevia to taste
dash of sea salt

Directions:

1. Split vanilla bean and use a sharp knife to scrape out the inside of the bean. Put scrapings in blender.
2. Combine all ingredients in blender and blend well.
3. Strain through a nut milk bag, or simply drink

Variation:

Omit the vanilla bean or use an alternative vanilla flavor. (I love toffee-flavored liquid stevia in this drink.)

Raw recipe

RICE MILK

I started experimenting with alternative milks because I couldn't find ones in the supermarket that were organic and/or not filled with sugar. This has become one of my absolute favorites. I do sometimes use rice that is from the refrigerator, but freshly cooked rice is best.

Ingredients:

- 1 vanilla bean
- 1 c. whole-grain rice (freshly cooked)
- 2 c. water
- stevia to taste
- dash of sea salt

Directions:

1. Split vanilla bean and use a sharp knife to scrape out the inside of the bean. Put scrapings in a blender.
2. Combine all ingredients in a blender and blend well.
3. Strain through a nut milk bag, or simply drink it as a thicker version. (The more rice you add, the thicker the milk will be.)

Variation

You can omit or use an alternative vanilla flavor for this milk. Toffee-flavored stevia (by Sweet Leaf) is one I sometimes use instead of the vanilla bean.

Note:

Honey or brown rice syrup works well as a sweetener.

Raw recipe

VEGAN EGG NOG

This is an easy version of egg nog. It makes a nice holiday drink!

Ingredients:

- 1½ c. vanilla-flavored, sweet almond, hazelnut, or rice milk
- 1 banana
- pinch of nutmeg
- a few drops stevia (optional)

Directions:

1. Place all ingredients in a blender and blend until creamy.

Note:

This recipe is easy to double.

Smoothies

Raw recipe

BASIC FRUIT SMOOTHIE

Fresh fruit is best for this recipe, but frozen works fine, too.

Ingredients:

1½ c. kombucha tea of choice or coconut water
1 or 2 bananas
1 apple, chopped (with skin)
1 c. berries (blueberries, strawberries, blackberries, raspberries, or a combination)
1 tsp. chia seeds

Directions:

1. Place all ingredients in a blender and blend well.

Variations:

1. Substitute pear or peach for apple.
2. Substitute cherries for berries.
3. Add a tablespoon of pomegranate seeds. (Buy them in the frozen food area of the grocery store.)
4. Add a tablespoon of pure, extra-virgin coconut oil for extra energy and nourishment.

Raw recipe

CHERRY-BANANA SMOOTHIE

This recipe is one of my seasonal favorites for August–September, when cherries are at their best. I use almond milk or whole-grain rice milk in this recipe. This recipe is for one large or two small servings.

Ingredients:

1 banana
1 c. fresh cherries, pitted
2 c. milk of choice
½ c. vanilla yogurt (optional)
1 T. maca root powder (optional)
1 T. raw, organic, pure, extra-virgin coconut oil
1 tsp. chia seeds
ice cubes for a colder smoothie (optional)

Directions:

1. Blend all ingredients in a blender until smooth.

Raw recipe

GREEN SMOOTHIE

The best drink I can suggest is this green smoothie, which is highly recommended for supreme health. It can help adjust pH balance and is used by many doctors to help diabetics keep blood sugar levels adjusted. It may sound unusual to you at first, but give it a try; you may be surprised by the taste.

It is best to make this drink in a good blender. (I recommend using something like the Breville blender or Vitamix because they can easily turn nuts, fruit, and vegetables to liquid.) This drink is rich in phytonutrients and Vitamin C. Try to drink it within 20 minutes of making it, as nutrients begin to dissipate after that time. Iron is more absorbable into the body when Vitamin C is present, so if you use spinach, this drink will be rich with Vitamin C and iron. A little-known fact is that spinach is 45% protein! In fact, the most protein-rich foods are leafy greens. The body does not turn protein like animal protein into protein in the body; it is the complex amino acid combinations in these greens that the body turns into protein in the body.

Ingredients:

1 c. leafy greens, torn into pieces (kale, lightly steamed spinach or beet greens, and fresh romaine, in any combination)
1 stalk celery, cut into pieces
½ cucumber, cut into chucks (with skin)
2 tsp. honey (optional)
1–2 T. lemon juice, freshly squeezed (or half a lemon if you really love citrus!)
2 c. coconut water or pure water (more water can be added to desired consistency)
dash of cinnamon (optional)
1 T. flax seed oil (cold-pressed) or ground flax seeds

Directions:

1. Put all ingredients in a blender and blend.

Variation:

Substitute dates (pitted and soaked in water to soften) for honey.

Raw recipe

PEACH SMOOTHIE

Flax seed oil and chia seeds both supply Omega 3 essential fatty acids.

Ingredients:

1 or 2 bananas
1¼ c. coconut water or milk (rice and almond milk are good choices)
2 peaches, cut in chunks
½ c. fresh pineapple, cut and drained
1 tsp. flax seed oil
1 tsp. chia seeds
a few ice cubes (optional)

Directions:

1. Blend all ingredients in a blender and enjoy!

Variations:

1. When using this as a breakfast drink for school or a meal replacement, it needs more fiber so you won't get hungry before lunch. I use Garden of Life brand fiber or I use psyllium husks. Just use a tiny bit, or it will expand when it gets wet and turn into a big glob that is hard to drink.
2. Add a splash of lime juice or a pitted date that has soaked for about 15 minutes to soften.

Raw recipe

SUPER CHOCOLATE POWER SMOOTHIE

Yes, you can have chocolate for breakfast and it will be healthy! Cacao is one of, if not the top anti-oxidant foods in the world. It is nutrient-dense. Note that if you're making this drink for someone who is diabetic, sweeten it with stevia or xylitol instead of using the dates.

Ingredients:

2½ c. almond milk
1 or 2 bananas
1 T. cacao powder or cacao nibs
2–3 dates, pitted and soaked in water for an hour or more
1 T. nut butter of choice (almond works well)
1 tsp. chia seeds

1T. extra-virgin, pure coconut oil
1 scoop protein powder
a few ice cubes (optional, but not recommended)

Directions:

1. Blend all ingredients well in a blender and enjoy!

Breakfast Foods

Raw recipe

CHIA SEED PUDDING

Chia seeds are from a plant that is a member of the mint family. They were used by the Aztecs and Mayans as a basic food source. Because they were so nutrient-dense, they were one of the main survival foods used by the warriors. They also had many medicinal uses. The Spanish banned the use of chia seeds after their conquest of Mexico, because the Aztecs used them in their religious worship and ceremonies. (The Spanish considered the Aztecs' religion pagan.) Chia seeds disappeared for a while, but they are making a comeback.

I use chia seeds in many of my recipes. They don't have much flavor, so they can easily be added to many recipes or dishes. I put chia seeds in water overnight in the refrigerator. When they are soaked in water or coconut water, they swell and become gelatinous, with a great, pudding-like consistency. I like to add this to my smoothies, peanut butter, cottage cheese, yogurt, salads, pancake mix, cookie mix, and breakfast dishes like oatmeal. I make my cashew crème and add it to the gelatinous chia mixture with a little fresh fruit for a wonderful breakfast dish or dessert.

These seeds are so full of high-soluble fiber that is easily used by the body, which makes eating them a wonderful way to reduce cravings, by helping you feel full and slowly releasing unrefined carbohydrates into your blood stream for natural energy. This makes them great for dieters or diabetics.

Start this recipe the day before you wish to serve it. This recipe is for one to two servings; it can easily be doubled.

Ingredients:

1 c. chia seeds
3½ c. purified water
fresh berries or sliced bananas (to add to the pudding; optional)
½ c. cashews
2 c. purified water
a few drops stevia (plain, toffee-flavored, or vanilla-flavored)

Directions for the pudding:

1. Soak chia seeds in 3½ c. water in a very large bowl (these seeds expand greatly) overnight in the refrigerator. The chia seeds get soft and expand, which makes the pudding. Add more water as necessary.

2. The next day, take pudding out of refrigerator and gently mix in berries or banana slices, if using.
3. Place chia pudding in individual serving bowls.

Directions for the cashew crème:

1. Soak cashews in 1 c. water overnight in the refrigerator. Pour off soaking water. The soaking water contains the phytic acid that we wanted to remove. The nuts are much more digestible when the phytic acid is removed. Then add 1 c. of clean, new water to blender.
2. Blend cashews and water with stevia, adding more water if you want it thinner. (I prefer it thick like a crème.)
3. Top each bowl of pudding with a dollop of cashew crème.

Note:

Sweet Leaf brand stevia comes in flavors like vanilla, orange, and toffee. They are really good for flavoring nut milks and crèmes. I usually find them at the healthy grocery store in the baking section or in the sweetener section.

COOKED OATMEAL

The flax seeds or chia seeds add Omega 3s to this dish. Enjoy this warm.

Ingredients:

2 c. water
1 c. steel-cut oats
1 tsp. honey
1 tsp. extra-virgin, pure coconut oil (optional)
sea salt to taste
¼–½ tsp. cinnamon
¼ c. raisins
2 T. freshly ground flax seeds or chia seeds
milk of choice (optional)

Directions:

1. Put water and oats in a pan and cook on a burner until boiling.
2. Stir continually until oats look a little creamy. This should be just a few minutes.
3. Remove from heat.
4. Add honey, coconut oil (if using), sea salt, cinnamon, raisins, and flax seeds or chia seeds.
5. Add milk, if using, to make creamier and less thick.

COTTAGE CHEESE WITH CINNAMON, HONEY, AND CHIA SEEDS

This is a slight variation of the flaxseed oil and cottage cheese recipe from the Dr. Johanna Budwig Diet. Dr. Budwig was one of Germany's top biochemists. She was also one of the best cancer researchers in Europe. Dr. Budwig was born in 1908 and lived to age 95. She was nominated for seven Nobel Prizes over a 50-year period, and Dr. Budwig had over a 90% success rate with her diet and protocol with all kinds of cancer patients. She developed great information about preventing and curing many diseases, including cancer, arthritis, multiple sclerosis, psoriasis, eczema, and acne. I got this recipe from the Budwig Diet Center website, which offers free downloads of Dr. Budwig's recipes. (I also like her mayonnaise recipe.) Learn more at www.budwigcenter.com/. I found out about Dr. Budwig and her research and recipes from a friend, and then I found Dr. Robert Willner, MD, PhD's The Cancer Solution. There is, however, a good deal of information on the Internet concerning Dr. Budwig and her work. (See the Resources.)

Cinnamon and honey are a delicious combination and have been found to have many healing benefits. This is a delicious way to have it in the morning.

Ingredients:

- 1 c. cottage cheese (organic)
- ½ tsp. cinnamon
- 2 tsp. honey
- 1 tsp. chia seeds
- ½ tsp. flax seed oil or freshly ground flax seeds
- 1 or 2 bananas, cut into chunks (optional)

Directions:

1. Combine all ingredients and enjoy!

Raw recipe

NANCY'S HOMEMADE GRANOLA

I had a tough time finding really good granola that doesn't contain sugar. Making your own is easy, if you have the right ingredients. I buy the highest-quality, organic, raw-food ingredients that I can find. The FDA requires that almonds be pasteurized. Pasteurization destroys the live enzymes in the nut, so if you want truly raw almonds, Google "nut farms" and "nut stores" to find sources of non-pasteurized and raw live nuts. They should be refrigerated.

Add things you like to this mixture, and diversify this recipe to suit your taste and the seasons. This recipe makes about 5 cups.

Ingredients:

- ½ c. almonds
- ½ c. walnuts
- ½ c. pumpkin seeds
- ½ c. sunflower seeds
- 1½ c. oats, fresh, raw, and preferably not contaminated with gluten at a silo or in transport
- ½ c. coconut, fresh or dried, and shredded
- ½ c. apricots, dried
- ½ c. cherries, dried
- ½ c. papaya, dried
- ½ c. dates, soaked in water until plump
- ¼ tsp. cinnamon
- 1 T. chia seeds or ground flax seeds
- fresh fruit (for example, banana, apple, or fresh berries; optional if eating immediately)

Directions:

1. Soak nuts for two hours to remove the phytic acid and make them more digestable.
2. Chop nuts and seeds.
3. Soak dried fruits for about an hour to soften them, and then chop.
4. Combine all ingredients in a bowl except fresh fruit, unless you are ready to eat it.

Notes:

1. Use a coffee bean grinder to grind nuts a little bit, but only pulse it. Don't grind it to a powder; let the nuts stay in pieces.
2. If you want to remove more of the phytic acid in the nuts, soak them in water for 12 to 18 hours and then dehydrate or put in the oven on low to dry them out.
3. Store this mixture in the refrigerator for a week or longer in the freezer. This mixture makes a decent trail mix, too, if it is dehydrated!
4. Serve this with a thick and rich nut milk or kefir.

RAW OATMEAL GRANOLA WITH YOGURT

This is a softer version of granola. You may want to start this the night before, in order to allow time for the oat flakes and chia seeds to soften and the nuts to be soaked. Soaking them breaks down the enzyme inhibitors and makes the oats, seeds and nuts more digestible. If you want the granola crunchier, make it fresh, do not soak the oats and seeds overnight, and use raw, unsoaked walnuts.

Ingredients:

½ c. raw oat flakes
2 T. chia seeds
1 c. water
1 c. yogurt
2 T. walnuts
½ tsp. cinnamon
2–4 dried (non-sulfured) apricots, chopped
1 c. raisins, softened by soaking in warm water at least 10 minutes

Directions:

1. Place oat flakes and chia seeds in water for an hour. Empty what liquid you can. Then soak oat flakes and chia seeds overnight in yogurt, in the refrigerator, to soften.
2. Soak walnuts for two to twelve hours in water to help them become more digestible.
3. Drain and chop walnuts.
4. Combine softened oats and chia seeds with all other ingredients. Let sit until it is room temperature, if you want it warm.

Variations:

1. Substitute kefir or a nut milk or hemp milk for yogurt.
2. Add a teaspoon of pure, extra-virgin coconut oil

SCRAMBLED EGGS

Buy organic, fresh eggs from chickens that are kept in open, fresh-air, sunny, green-grass environments. You may want to find a local farmer you can trust from whom you can buy your eggs.

The ingredients listed here are for one serving.

Ingredients:

2–3 eggs
2 T. milk of choice
1 or 2 T. coconut oil
sea salt to taste
pepper to taste

Directions:

1. Beat eggs in a bowl with milk.
2. Heat oil in a skillet over medium heat.
3. Put eggs in the skillet and stir until eggs are cooked to your liking.
4. Add salt and pepper to taste.

Note:

Use a little more oil (a teaspoon or more) if you are cooking more than four eggs.

Variations:

1. Add some chopped onion, tomatoes, and/or mushrooms.
2. Make this as an omelet: Don't stir eggs when they are in the pan. Let cook, and then gently fold over and slide out of the pan onto a plate.

Lunch, Travel, and Snack Foods

If you are like me, you are always in need of some kind of food to take with you, whether it is for school, work, or travel. Having a good plan that is easy, healthy, low-cost, and delicious makes those days seem so much better. Some of my favorite things to make are pita sandwiches, crackers with a protein-rich salad, salad topped with beans and sprouts, or simply a variety of cut-up veggies to snack on all day. Nuts, whole-grain crackers, and bite-sized fruit are also great snacks. I usually take time on Sunday to cut up veggies or to cook beans I am going to eat during the week. I make a large amount of beans and either use them all week or freeze them for the next week. Making a couple of different types of beans provides some variety. I also fill baggies or travel cups with nuts, seeds, and dried fruits so I can grab them quickly in the morning when I am in a hurry. For a simple sandwich, try using pita bread. Pitas are good because they hold fillings well and are not too messy. There are some wonderful whole-grain pita breads at many grocery stores. Look for them in the freezer section or with the breads.

Raw recipe, gluten free

ENERGY PROTEIN BARS

These are really healthy, easy, and delicious!

Ingredients:

1 cup raisins

½ c. almonds, soaked at least 12 hours in water. Discard the water the almonds in which they were soaking.

4 medjool dates, pitted and soaked at least 1 hour in a little bit of water. Save two tablespoons of this water to add to the food processing mixture.

2 T. Date soaking water or plain water.

¼ c. freshly ground flax seeds

½ dropper of liquid stevia (plain or toffee flavor)

2 c. (gluten free) steel cut oats

1 T. chia seeds

3 T. raw, organic sunflower seeds and or pumpkin seeds or a mixture of both.

1 c. vanilla flavored Garden of Life Protein Powder or a vanilla flavored protein powder of your choice

¼ tsp. sea salt

1 T. extra-virgin, pure coconut oil

Directions:

1. Combine all ingredients in a food processor and pulse the mixture until it creates a dough like consistency. If it's too thick, add a little more water. If it's too thin, then add a little more oats until it is thicker.
2. Line a 2" deep glass or ceramic baking dish with wax paper and then spread out the mixture in the baking dish about 1/2-inch thick.
3. Place in refrigerator for at least an hour to firm. If you want it firmer, place it in the freezer.
4. Using the wax paper, you can lift the bars out of the dish and place it on a cutting board. Remove the wax paper and slice into bars.

Notes:

1. Soaking almonds makes them easier to digest.
2. Store bars in an airtight container wrapped in plastic wrap or parchment paper. Store in the refrigerator for added freshness.
3. Oats are naturally gluten free, but they must be stored and transported in gluten free containers, in order for them to be labeled gluten free.

Raw recipe

KALE CHIPS

This delicious, nutritious, fun, and easy snack or side dish is made with a dehydrator.

Kale chips are crispy, thin chips made from fresh kale. Kale shrinks a great deal, so make one bunch for each person.

Ingredients:

1 bunch fresh kale per person
extra-virgin olive oil (about 1 T.)
honey (about ½ tsp.; optional)
sea salt (about ¼ tsp.)
mesquite powder (about ¼ tsp.)
cinnamon (about ¼ tsp.)

Directions:

1. Cut kale in approximately 2-inch-square pieces.
2. Rub each piece with extra-virgin olive oil.
3. Drizzle with honey, if using.
4. Sprinkle lightly with all of the seasonings.
5. Dehydrate about 10 hours until crispy.

Notes:

1. I love honey on my kale chips. It makes them sweet, as well as spicy and salty.
2. I usually dehydrate chips overnight.
3. Store kale chips in an airtight container so they will keep for a few days.

Raw recipe

MUSHROOM NIBBLES

I love mushrooms, and I make these quick and easy nibbles all the time. I serve these as a quick bite for lunch or a snack. They are terrific as appetizers and/or a side dish. Serve them warm.

Ingredients:

10 or more button or small cap mushrooms
enough soy sauce (organic and unpasteurized) to cover the mushrooms

¼ c. Pesto (recipe on page 227)
¼ c. raw, organic goat cheese (optional)

Directions:

1. Brush off mushrooms and remove stems.
2. Soak mushrooms in soy sauce two hours or overnight.
3. After soaking, place mushrooms in a baking dish.
4. Fill mushrooms with pesto and top with a dab of goat cheese, if using.
5. Warm mushrooms in an oven, toaster oven, or warming drawer.

Notes:

I soak the stems, too, chop them, and save them for use in other recipes.

When warming, keep the temperature under 118 degrees to keep the enzymes alive.

Raw recipe

NORI ROLLS WITH NUT PÂTÉ

These are easy and delicious. The first time I made this recipe was when I needed a quick lunch to take with me on an airplane. This is a great finger food and makes a terrific appetizer.

Ingredients:

2–3 nori sheets
1 cup Nut Pâté (thick; recipe on page 178)
1–2 avocados, sliced
1 carrot, julienned
½ c. sprouts (sunflower or broccoli)
½ c. soy sauce (unpasteurized, organic; for dipping)
¼ c. wasabi (optional)
¼ c. pickled ginger (optional)

Directions:

1. Lay out nori sheets (shiny side down) on a flat surface or a bamboo (sushi) mat (that can roll up).
2. Spread a thick layer of Nut Pâté on a middle section of each nori sheet all the way across, about an inch tall, leaving about a half-inch border from the outside edge.
3. Spread slices of avocado over Nut Pâté, staying inside the edge by about a half-inch. (Lay them horizontally.)

4. Place carrots in a thick layer on the sheets in a horizontal position from you.
5. Lay an even layer of sprouts across the carrots and avocado.
6. Take the end of the nori sheet right in front of you and start rolling it, away from you.
7. Seal the final edge with a little water to make it stick.
8. Slice this across the roll into about 1-inch-thick rolls.
9. Dip pieces in soy sauce and enjoy with wasabi and/or pickled ginger, if using.

Notes:

1. The nori will cut easier if you use a very sharp knife.
2. Avocado is one of the two main ingredients in the recipe, so use a half or a whole avocado for each roll.

Raw recipe

NUT PÂTÉ

This is an easy, rich, and savory snack or appetizer.

I like to use this as a filling for my Nori Rolls with Nut Pâté (recipe on page 177). You could also serve this with crackers or with chopped vegetables as a dip.

Ingredients:

1 c. walnuts, soaked 12 to 18 hours in water in the refrigerator
1 c. pecans, soaked 12 to 18 hours in water in the refrigerator
1 red bell pepper, chopped
2 stalks celery, chopped
2 T. lemon juice (fresh)
1 tsp. sensational sea salt (see resources page: 299)
dash of mesquite powder (optional)

Directions:

1. Combine all ingredients in a food processor.
2. Add a little water if necessary.

PITA SANDWICH

I like many different kinds of pita sandwiches, but here is an all-time satisfying one to try. You can make this pita sandwich quickly. When you use avocado, it is better to eat the pita sandwich right away. If you won't be eating this right away, wrap it tightly to keep out the air, or the avocado can turn dark. Because of the nature of avocado, you can mash the avocado with a little lemon juice to help it stay fresher and greener longer.

Ingredients:

1 whole-grain pita
1 avocado, sliced
1/4 c. black beans, cooked
1 small tomato, sliced
3 T. sprouts
pinch of sea salt
1–2 slices mozzarella cheese (optional)

Directions:

1. Layer ingredients inpita bread.

Variations:

1. Substitute goat cheese for mozzarella.
2. Add some chopped onion.
3. Add a few leaves of spinach.
4. Substitute kidney beans for black beans.
5. Substitute mustard or mayonnaise for avocado.

ROASTED CHESTNUTS

When I was living in London, I always loved to smell the roasted chestnuts sold on street corners during the winter months. When they are roasted, they fill the air with a wonderful aroma. Rich and delicious chestnuts are used to add flavor to many European winter dishes.

Chestnuts can be roasted over an open fire or fireplace in a large, long-handled frying pan.

Serve these as a snack or appetizer.

Ingredients:

whole chestnuts

Directions:

1. Soak chestnuts about an hour in water or vegetable broth, then drain.
2. Score the bottom of each nut with an X to let the steam escape. (This also makes them easier to peel when they are finished cooking.)

3. Place nuts in a frying pan and cook over open fire about 20 minutes.
4. After chestnuts have cooled down a little, peel them.

Note:

If you don't have an open fire, place nuts on a cookie sheet and bake them in a preheated, 425-degree oven for about 20 minutes.

SPROUT SANDWICH

This is a yummy sandwich I have been enjoying since I was a teenager. I grew up eating sprouts and butter sandwiches. Now I like to add some avocado, but I still love the buttery flavor, so sometimes I add a little bit of ghee to the sandwich as well.

You can wrap this tightly if you are going to take this sandwich with you, or eat it right away! If you aren't eating it right away, you may want to put it in the refrigerator until you are ready to eat it.

Ingredients:

1 avocado
1 T. softened ghee (optional)
2 slices soft, whole-grain bread of choice
sea salt
½–1 c. sprouts of choice (alfalfa, broccoli, etc.)

Directions:

1. Mash avocado.
2. Spread ghee on bread.
3. Spread some avocado on each slice of bread.
4. Sprinkle with sea salt.
5. Heap sprouts on top of avocado.
6. Cover with the other piece of bread.

Raw recipe

TABBOULEH

This is a Middle Eastern cold salad. It can be very refreshing and delicious on a hot summer day. Quinoa is a complete amino acid complex food, so this makes a very nutritious and satisfying dish. Parsley is one of the few foods that contain Vitamin D. You need to start this salad a day or two ahead of time. Tabbouleh can be refrigerated for two to three days, so you can make it ahead of time and serve easily when entertaining or for a meal on the go. It goes well with whole-grain breads, pita, or crackers.

Ingredients:

- 2 c. quinoa, soaked overnight and then spouted for 1–2 days (or cooked in water until tender)
- 2 large tomatoes, diced
- 1 c. parsley (fresh), chopped
- 1 red bell pepper, diced
- 3 small green onions, diced
- 1 large cucumber, diced
- ½ c. extra-virgin olive oil
- ½ c. lemon juice (fresh)
- sea salt to taste
- 1 tsp. soy sauce (optional)

Directions:

1. In a large bowl, combine all ingredients and toss well.
2. Chill overnight.

Notes:

1. If you're soaking/sprouting the quinoa: Soak quinoa overnight. Put it in a strainer with a kitchen hand towel placed over it, so it is kept out of the light. Allow it to sprout for a day.
2. I always use red or yellow bell peppers for this recipe. (Green bell peppers are not fully ripe.)

Raw recipe

TRAIL MIX

I had trouble finding a trail mix that I liked that didn't have some sort of sugar added to it, so I decided to make my own. Trail mix is wonderful to keep on hand for traveling, a daily running-around emergency food, or a snack at the office or school.

If you love chocolate, add it to this mix and it will meld right in! If you just want a hint of cacao, use cacao powder instead of cacao nibs.

Ingredients:

- ½ c. pecans
- ½ c. pine nuts
- ½ c. almonds
- ½ c. walnuts
- ½ c. pistachios
- ½ c. pumpkin seeds
- ½ c. sunflower seeds

½ c. coconut (fresh or dried), shredded
½ c. apricots (dried), chopped
1 c. cherries (dried), chopped
½ c. raisins
½ c. medjool dates
½ c. papaya (dried), chopped
¼ tsp. sea salt
1/8 c. cacao nibs or powder (optional)

Directions:

1. Soak all nuts 12 hours in water, and then let them dry well. Dry them in a dehydrator for a few hours, if you have one. If you don't, spread them on a cookie sheet and let them sit in a very dry, slightly warm oven (less than 118 degrees) at least an hour.
2. Combine all ingredients in a bowl.

Notes:

1. Soaking the nuts makes them more digestible and helps eliminate the phytic acid and enzyme inhibitors.
2. Store this in an airtight glass container, or put it into small containers ready to grab quickly. Keep it in the refrigerator, so it will stay fresh longer.
3. Eat this mixture within a week. Since the nuts are soaked, they won't last as long. You can freeze it and then thaw out what you need.

Main Dishes

BASIC STIR FRY

Stir fry or wok cooking is a healthy way to make a great meal! All you really need for this are some peanut or sesame seed oil, some seitan (wheat meat) or mushrooms, and some of your favorite vegetables (sliced or chopped). When you cook, simply keep the foods moving so everything gets heated and cooked without getting overcooked. I love adding different sauces to the stir fry in order to have more variety in my meals. One day I might add a black bean sauce, and the next day a hoisin sauce or even a sweet and sour sauce. You can even make your own sauce, or use a low-salt soy sauce or miso. When you are buying a pre-made sauce, look at the ingredient list for sugar, salt, fats, chemical additives (which can be disguised under names like "natural flavorings" and "natural spices"), and calories. The first four or five ingredients are probably the most important ones to be aware of, but take the time to read them all.

This recipe allows you to change the sauce whenever you want to have a new taste sensation. The stir fry can be very light, heart- and weight-healthy, yet savory and delicious. Change the type of vegetables and buy the best in season, and you can have an easy, home-cooked meal without much prep time or clean-up time.

Serve this dish warm, with a side of whole-grain rice.

Ingredients:

2 T. sesame oil or peanut oil
1 lb. seitan, cut in ½-inch pieces
1 tsp. miso
2 T. water
¼ c. scallions, finely chopped
½ c. mushrooms, sliced
½ c. water chestnuts
½ c. snow peas
2 cloves garlic, minced
2 carrots, julienned
¼ c. vegetable broth

Directions:

1. Heat oil in stainless steel skillet or wok.
2. Add seitan and sauté rapidly, turning pieces constantly to cook evenly. When done, remove from heat and keep warm.
3. Dissolve miso in water.
4. Add remaining ingredients to the pan and stir fry 3–5 minutes.
5. Return seitan to pan, stir a moment, and remove from heat.

Variations:

1. Substitute tempeh for seitan.
2. Add chow mein noodles or chopped cilantro to the final dish as a garnish.
3. Add cooked lo mein or rice noodles.
4. Omit seitan completely and increase mushrooms. Cook vegetables and mushrooms with oil for about 3 minutes before adding miso water.

BEAN AND CHEESE ENCHILADAS

I used to make these for my children when they came home hungry from school, or for wonderful lunches and/or dinners. They liked them plain, but you can serve pico de gallo or salsa with this dish. This was one of their favorite meals. Serve warm.

I am listing the ingredients for one serving. Use these amounts for each enchilada you're making.

Ingredients:

1 T. extra-virgin, pure coconut oil
1 whole-grain, organic tortilla
¼ c. cheese of choice, grated
¼ c. warm baked beans

Directions:

1. Heat a grill or large fry pan.
2. Put a little oil on the griddle.
3. Place tortilla on griddle and warm. Turn tortilla over and coat with coconut oil.
4. Sprinkle grated cheese on the middle of the tortilla, and then spread the warm beans over it.
5. As soon as cheese starts to melt, fold one side over the middle, take the opposite side and fold it over the middle, and slide the folded-over enchilada off the griddle onto a plate.
6. Serve warm.

Notes:

1. Play with the amount of beans or cheese you want in each tortilla.
2. Any variety beans will work, but kidney beans and black beans work well.

Variation:

Add some chopped tomato, chopped onions, or chopped jalapeño.

BEAN LASAGNA

This is hearty, cost-effective meal. Lasagna is easy to freeze and reheat. I sometimes make two at a time, and freeze one. Bake this in a 13 x 9 x 2 dish that's deep enough for the layers of the lasagna.

Serve this with crusty, hot, whole-grain bread and a salad.

Ingredients:

- 8 oz. whole-grain lasagna noodles
- 2 eggs
- 1 16-oz. container ricotta cheese
- 2 c. mozzarella cheese, grated
- 1 c. Parmesan cheese, grated
- ¾ tsp. sea salt
- ¾ tsp. black pepper
- 1 c. onion, chopped
- 1 T. extra-virgin, pure coconut oil
- 2 c. great northern or pinto beans (cooked)
- 2 cloves garlic, minced
- 1 tsp. oregano
- 1 tsp. basil
- 3 c. tomato sauce

Directions:

1. Preheat oven to 375 degrees.
2. Boil a pot of water and cook lasagna noodles until al dente. (This means they are soft, but not too soft; there is a tiny bit of hardness to them.) When they are al dente, remove from heat, drain, and set aside.
3. Beat eggs.
4. Combine eggs with ricotta cheese, mozzarella cheese, ¼ cup of the Parmesan cheese, ½ teaspoon of the sea salt, and ½ teaspoon of the black pepper. Set aside.
5. Sauté onion in a very large skillet or heavy-bottomed pot with coconut oil until almost translucent.
6. Add cooked beans, minced garlic, remaining ¼ teaspoon of salt, remaining ¼ teaspoon of pepper, oregano, and basil, and sauté a few more minutes.
7. Add tomato sauce and stir a few more minutes until combined well.
8. In the baking dish, layer the lasagna: Start with 1/3 of the bean-tomato mixture, followed by a layer of noodles, then half of the cheese mixture evenly. Repeat the layers. Finish with the last 1/3 of the bean-tomato mixture and sprinkle the remaining Parmesan cheese over the top.
9. Bake 30 minutes.

Notes:

1. I love to use roasted tomato sauce in this recipe. Muir Glen has a wonderful roasted tomato sauce that comes in a glass jar. (See the Resources.)

2. It is easy to use a whole grain, gluten free lasagna noodle. See resources for gluten free noodles.

BROCCOLI LASAGNA

I love lasagna, and this is one of my favorite dishes to serve when I have company. It is easy to make ahead of time, refrigerate, and then reheat for the dinner. This looks like a complicated recipe, but it is actually pretty easy. You can buy frozen broccoli and spinach and thaw them, and buy cheeses already grated. This will make the preparation a little easier. I usually make two or three lasagnas at a time and freeze them. Having these lasagnas on hand makes everything about entertaining so easy. I have had many of my meat-eating friends tell me that they absolutely love this lasagna, so it has passed the "non-vegetarian dinner guest test" at my home (and this is in Texas, where that test can be a tough one!). Bake this lasagna in a 13 x 9 x 2 dish that's deep enough for the layers of the lasagna.

Serve this with salad and crusty, whole-grain bread.

Ingredients:

dash of cayenne pepper
pinch of garlic salt
pinch of onion powder
1/8 tsp. basil (dried)
1/8 tsp. thyme (dried)
1/8 tsp. parsley (dried)
1/8 tsp. savory (dried)
1/8 tsp. sage (dried)
1 tsp. miso
¼ c. water
8 oz. whole-grain lasagna noodles
2 eggs
1 16-oz. container ricotta cheese
2 c. mozzarella cheese, grated
1 c. Parmesan cheese, grated
½ c. parsley (fresh), chopped
¼ tsp. sea salt
¼ tsp. black pepper
1 c. onion, chopped
1 T. extra-virgin, pure coconut oil
1 c. mushrooms, sliced
2 cloves garlic, minced
2 c. broccoli, chopped
½ c. spinach, chopped
3 c. tomato sauce

Directions:

1. Preheat oven to 375 degrees.
2. Combine cayenne pepper, garlic salt, onion powder, basil, thyme, dried parsley, savory, and sage. Set aside.
3. Dissolve miso in the ¼ c. of water. Set aside.
4. Boil a pot of water and cook lasagna noodles until al dente. (This means they are soft, but not too soft; there is a tiny bit of hardness to them.) When they are al dente, remove from heat, drain, and set aside.
5. Beat eggs.
6. Combine eggs with ricotta cheese, mozzarella cheese, ¼ cup of the Parmesan cheese, fresh parsley, the herb combination (cayenne, garlic salt, onion powder, basil, thyme, parsley, savory and sage that was set aside) salt, and pepper. Set aside.
7. Sauté onions in a large skillet with coconut oil until almost translucent, then add the mushrooms and minced garlic and sauté a few more minutes.
8. Add miso water to the skillet with onion mixture carefully, so it doesn't splatter.
9. Quickly add chopped broccoli and spinach, and sauté a few minutes. Remove from heat and set aside.
10. In the baking dish, layer the lasagna: Start with 1/3 of the tomato sauce, followed by a layer of noodles, then half of the cheese mixture evenly, then half of the vegetable mixture evenly. Repeat the layers. Finish with the last 1/3 of the tomato sauce and sprinkle the remaining Parmesan cheese over the top.
11. Bake 25 to 30 minutes.

Notes:

1. I love to use roasted tomato sauce with this recipe.
2. Garlic salt can be found in the spice area at the grocery store. You can also simply mince some garlic and add it to some sea salt to make your own.
3. It is easy to use gluten free lasagna noodles in this recipe. For gluten free noodles, see resources.

GIBBONS BURGER

This is an old recipe my father invented. I have absolutely no idea why my father called it a burger! It is an open sandwich that is nothing like a burger, but that is the name it has been called for decades. It's a family favorite. My father used white French bread, but I substitute whole-grain French bread. Any whole-grain bread will do, but a thick piece, like half of a hamburger bun, works best. This is the recipe for one sandwich. Use these amounts for each sandwich you make.

Ingredients:

1 piece thickly sliced whole-grain bread
¼ c. red bell pepper, washed and thinly (about ¼ inch) sliced into long strips
butter or ghee
1 or 2 fresh garlic cloves, minced
sprinkle of sea salt (to taste)
¼ c. cheddar cheese (raw organic is best) sliced into thin (about ¼-inch) strips

Directions:

1. Place bread on a baking sheet or a toaster oven rack.
2. Place bell pepper strips on bread.
3. Melt butter with garlic in it.
4. Drizzle melted garlic butter over bread and pepper slices.
5. Sprinkle with sea salt
6. Lay slices of cheese evenly on top.
7. Place in toaster oven or oven to broil until cheese is melted.

Variation:

Substitute garlic salt for fresh garlic.

GIBBONS'S ROASTED VEGETABLE PITA SANDWICH

My son loves to make these delicious sandwiches during the summer. This recipe makes one serving.

Ingredients:

1 whole-grain pita bread, warmed
½ zucchini, thinly sliced lengthwise
¼ c. red or yellow bell peppers, thinly sliced

1 carrot, thinly sliced
½ c. hummus

Directions:

1. Preheat oven to 475 degrees.
2. Spread zucchini, peppers, and carrot slices on a roasting pan and place in oven.
3. Roast vegetables 10 to 15 minutes, until they are slightly soft and warm.
4. Spread hummus in the warm pita bread.
5. Lay slices of roasted vegetables in layers inside warm pita bread on top of hummus.

Variations:

1. Coat vegetables with a little coconut oil and sea salt before roasting for a richer and moister flavor.
2. Substitute grilled vegetables for roasted vegetables.
3. Substitute mayonnaise or sliced avocado for hummus.

MEXICAN BLACK BEAN AND SPINACH PIZZA

This is a favorite recipe of my niece Claire and her husband, Stefan.

Ingredients:

1 10-oz. whole-grain pizza crust
1 can black beans, rinsed and drained
2/3 c. chopped onion
1 tsp. ground cumin
1 tsp. chili powder
1 garlic clove, minced
½ c. bottled salsa
½ of 10-oz. package frozen spinach, thawed, drained, and dried
2 T. chopped fresh cilantro
1 small can diced green chiles
½ tsp. hot sauce
½ c. Monterey Jack cheese, grated
½ c. reduced-fat sharp cheddar, grated

Directions:

1. Preheat oven to 375 degrees.
2. Place pizza crust on a baking sheet; bake 5 minutes or until crisp.

3. Mash beans with a fork; combine beans, onion, cumin, chili powder, and garlic in a medium bowl, stirring to combine.
4. Spread bean mixture over crust, leaving a 1-inch border.
5. Spoon salsa evenly over bean mixture; top with spinach, cilantro, and green chiles. Drizzle with hot sauce; sprinkle with cheeses.
6. Bake 15 minutes or until crust is lightly browned.

Variations:

1. Brush olive oil on crust and sprinkle some freshly grated Parmesan cheese before toasting in a 450-degree oven for 5 to 7 minutes.
2. Substitute diced jalapeno for (or in addition to) green chiles.

PORTOBELLO MUSHROOM BURGER

This is one of my favorite savory meals. I have made this for many non-vegetarian Texans with success, much to their surprise! The quantities here are enough for one person. You can make as many sandwiches as you want by adjusting the ingredient amounts accordingly.

Ingredients:

1 large portobello mushroom
3 T. soy sauce
1 whole-grain hamburger bun or bread
¼ c. goat cheese, sliced
a few leaves romaine lettuce

Directions:

1. Brush off mushroom and remove stem.
2. Soak in soy sauce at least five minutes (20 minutes is better).
3. Bake at 350 degrees or broil in an oven, just until thoroughly warm, making sure it is moist with the soy sauce.
4. Warm or toast bun.
5. Place cheese on top of mushroom and leave in oven just a couple of minutes.
6. Remove mushroom from oven and place on bun.
7. Place lettuce on top of cheese.
8. Place top bun on sandwich.

Variations:

1. Slice and add avocado.
2. Add mayonnaise. Mayonnaise is really delicious with this sandwich.

POTATO, BROCCOLI, AND BEAN STEW

I love broccoli and potatoes together. Add beans, and you have a rich and hearty dish. This is actually quite easy; you can use canned beans if you need to. I like to use white northern beans, but kidney beans will work as well.

This is a nice meal to serve when entertaining because you can make it ahead of time and warm it up when you're ready to serve. Serve this with a salad and crusty, whole-grain bread. Inexpensive, satisfying, easy, and full of nutrition—this meal is hard to beat.

Ingredients:

1½ lb. potatoes, cut into 2-inch cubes
1 T. extra-virgin, pure coconut oil
½ tsp. sea salt
10 c. water
2 c. northern white beans (cooked)
2 c. broccoli, cut in ½- to 1-inch pieces
4 garlic cloves, minced
1 tsp. red pepper flakes
¼ tsp. pepper, freshly ground

Directions:

1. Cook potatoes, coconut oil, and sea salt in the water until potatoes are just tender. (This can take anywhere from 25 to 40 minutes.)
2. Add beans, broccoli, garlic, red pepper flakes, and pepper. Stir for a few minutes, and then simmer about 10 minutes, stirring occasionally (so that nothing burns).
3. Serve warm.

Note:

Yukon gold, purple, and sweet potatoes are all good choices.

QUICK AND EASY PIZZA

This pizza makes a great lunch, dinner, or after-school snack. Enjoy!

Truffle oil is one of my favorite oils to use in recipes. It makes dishes really rich and unique.

Ingredients:

1 whole-grain, ready-to-use pizza crust
1½ c. shredded organic mozzarella cheese
½ c. tomatoes, thinly sliced (¼-inch-thick)

1 clove garlic, minced
¼ c. red or sweet onion, thinly sliced
a few leaves basil (fresh), chopped
½ tsp. truffle oil (optional)

Directions:

1. Preheat oven to 375 degrees.
2. Place cheese evenly on the top of the pizza crust or bread.
3. Spread tomatoes on top.
4. Put garlic, onion, and basil evenly on top of the tomatoes.
5. Drizzle truffle oil, if using, over the top for an extra-special taste!
6. Place pizza in oven until crust is baked, or the cheese is melted and slightly brown on the edges

Variation:

Use a whole-grain pita, an English muffin, or simply a thick slice of whole-grain bread instead of pizza crust. Adjust ingredient amounts as needed.

SEITAN POT PIE

This easy recipe comes from my mom's friend Evelyn Bridges. I changed her recipe to make it vegetarian. Use any milk you prefer in this recipe. I usually use rice milk.

Ingredients:

3 c. seitan, cut in ½-inch chunks
¾ c. carrots, sliced and parboiled
1 14.5-oz. can peas (or 1 c. fresh)
sea salt to taste
pepper to taste
1 14.5-oz. can cream of celery soup
1½ c. milk
1½ c. vegetable broth
1½ c. Texas Biscuits recipe dough (recipe on page 257), mixed and ready to bake
½ stick butter, melted, or ghee

Directions:

1. Preheat oven to 375 degrees.

2. Put seitan in the bottom of a 2-quart casserole dish.
3. Sprinkle carrots and then peas over seitan.
4. Sprinkle with salt and pepper.
5. Mix soup, milk, and broth together, and pour over seitan and vegetables.
6. Gently spoon Texas Biscuit dough on top.
7. Drizzle butter or ghee over the top of all.
8. Bake, uncovered, one hour or until hot and bubbly.

Note:

If there's extra dough, use it to make a few biscuits.

Variation:

Substitute extra-virgin, pure coconut oil for butter.

SEITAN STROGANOFF

This is a vegetarian variation of one of my mother's recipes. Seitan is of Japanese origin and is a rich source of vegetable protein. It is made from wheat flour and is known as "wheat meat." It has a delicious flavor. Seitan contains an equal amount of protein as an equal-sized portion of sirloin beef. Seitan has no cholesterol or saturated fat. Seitan has twice the amount of protein as an equal-sized portion of tofu. Seitan can be stored in a broth for seven to 10 days in the refrigerator. It will keep for several months in a freezer.

Serve this recipe over hot, whole-grain rice.

Ingredients:

1 lb. seitan, cut in ¾-inch cubes
½ c. mushrooms
sea salt to taste
pepper to taste
¾ c. whole-grain flour
3-4 T. extra-virgin, pure coconut oil
1 c. onion, chopped
1 clove garlic, minced
1 14.5-oz. can mushroom sauce or mushroom soup
1 T. Worcestershire sauce
1 c. water
1 pint sour cream

Directions:

1. Season seitan and mushrooms with salt and pepper, dip in flour, and sauté in hot coconut oil until lightly brown.

2. Add onion, garlic, mushroom sauce, and Worcestershire sauce.
3. Add water and simmer, covered, about half an hour or until seitan is tender. (You may need to add a little more water.)
4. Remove from heat and stir in sour cream.

Variation:

Substitute tempeh for seitan.

SHISH KEBABS

Traditionally, a shish kebab is meat cooked on a stick. Shish kebab actually means "roast meat." The shish kebab was developed by nomadic peoples who once inhabited the area around present-day Turkey. Today variations of the dish exist in almost every culture. In Asia they are called satay and are usually served with a dipping sauce. The French call them brochettes, meaning skewers. Whatever the terminology, this dish is easy to prepare, serve, and eat.

Shish kebabs make a perfect dinner whether you are entertaining, want an easy dinner at home, or even are camping. They can be prepared in advance and assembled fairly quickly. Allow the seitan and/or mushrooms to marinate for at least an hour in the refrigerator to absorb the flavor. The marinade can be as easy as your favorite teriyaki sauce, Italian salad dressing, or barbeque sauce—or you can be creative and mix and match fruit juices, hot sauces, herbs, and spices to create your own signature marinade.

Dinner on a stick is especially fun as a hands-on cooking and eating experience for kids. The main utensil needed will be metal or wood skewers. Always soak wood skewers 20–30 minutes, and then dry off any excess water before assembling; this keeps them from catching fire while cooking.

This is a great vegetarian dish that can fill that craving for a meat type of food. When I first became a vegetarian, I missed the chewing, the barbecue sauce, and the texture of meat. Wheat meat, or seitan, really can be extremely delicious. Seitan is of Japanese origin and is one of the richest sources of vegetarian protein. It is equal in protein to the equivalent portion of sirloin beef. Seitan, however, has no cholesterol or saturated fat. It has less than half the amount of calories of the equivalent-sized portion of meat.

I prefer to use seitan instead of tofu. Seitan has twice the amount of protein as tofu, and I like the texture better. Mushrooms are also a wonderful, hearty substitute for meat. I have combined the two here to make a rich, hearty meal. Mix in a variety of flavors and colors by adding different fruits and vegetables. When everything comes together, you will have a beautiful, fun, and delicious meal!

This recipe will fill approximately 25 8-inch skewers.

Ingredients:

- 1 lb. seitan, cut in 1½-inch cubes
- 1 lb. mushrooms, stems removed
- 1 c. or more teriyaki sauce
- extra-virgin, pure coconut oil
- 1 large red onion, cut in 1- to 1½-inch squares
- 2 zucchini, thickly sliced
- 1½ c. cherry tomatoes, whole
- 1 pineapple, cut into 1-inch cubes
- salt to taste (optional)
- pepper to taste (optional)

Directions:

1. Place seitan and mushrooms in a large zip-top bag with enough teriyaki sauce to completely cover them. Refrigerate an hour or two, turning bag over every once in a while to make sure seitan and mushrooms are thoroughly marinated.
2. If you are using a grill, start the fire. (Skewers can also be broiled or baked in the oven or grilled on an electric indoor grill.)
3. If using wood skewers, soak in water 20–30 minutes, then dry.
4. Rub skewers with coconut oil.
5. Assemble skewers with seitan, mushrooms, onion, zucchini, tomatoes, and pineapple.
6. Put skewers in a large zip-top baggie with teriyaki sauce and keep in the refrigerator until time to cook.
7. Bake, broil, or grill shish kebabs over medium heat for about 10 minutes, or until seitan is done to your liking, turning kebabs every few minutes. Watch to make sure they don't burn.
8. Season with salt and pepper to taste.

Notes:

1. Teriyaki sauce is rather salty. Because of this, you may not need to add additional salt and pepper to this recipe.
2. You can assemble skewers in advance.
3. For a nice glaze, and to keep kebabs more moist, brush them

with marinade while cooking.

Variation:

Make your own marinade for this dish. Using olive oil, garlic, herbs, soy sauce, and a little honey or brown rice syrup, you can make a very nice marinade of your own creation.

SPINACH QUICHE

I love to make quiche. It is easy to make and easy to store, and it can be eaten warm or cold. I use a variety of ingredients for the filling. This is my basic recipe.

I use a pre-made, whole-grain crust from the frozen food department at my grocery store. This is an easy dish to prepare for company or parties.

Ingredients:

1 whole-grain pie crust
½ onion, chopped
1 tsp. extra-virgin, pure coconut oil
1¼ c. fresh spinach
1 c. milk
3 eggs, well beaten
1 tsp. parsley, dried or freshly minced
½ tsp. chives, dried or freshly minced
3 T. butter, melted
1 T. mustard
1 c. cheddar cheese, grated
½ c. mozzarella cheese, grated
½ tsp. sea salt
¼ tsp. pepper

Directions:

1. Preheat oven to 350 degrees.
2. Pierce pie crust with the tines of a fork to make a few air holes in the crust, so it won't make air-filled bubbles when it is cooking.
3. Bake crust empty for about 8 minutes. Remove from oven to cool slightly.
4. Sauté onion and coconut oil until onion is slightly soft and translucent.
5. Add spinach and sauté for just a moment before removing from heat.
6. Mix together milk, eggs, parsley, chives, and butter, and set aside.
7. Spread mustard evenly around the base of the pie crust.
8. Spread onions and spinach evenly around the pie crust over mustard.
9. Combine cheeses and sprinkle over spinach.
10. Sprinkle salt and pepper over spinach and cheese.
11. Pour milk, egg, and butter mixture over spinach and cheese.
12. Bake 30–45 minutes, until top is golden brown and the pie seems

firm. (You can also stick a toothpick in the center to see if it comes out clean.)

13. Let quiche sit for at least five minutes before cutting.

Note:

I like to use spicy hot mustard.

Variations:

1. Substitute asparagus or broccoli for spinach.
2. Use different cheeses like Monterey Jack. I like to use a chipotle cranberry cheese to give my quiche a little kick!
3. Substitute almond milk or goat milk for cow milk.

TACO SALAD

Sometimes I just feel like something crunchy, salty, and Mexican! Growing up in Texas meant having a true appreciation for Mexican food. When I became a vegetarian, it became a little more challenging; many chips, salsas, and beans have meat broth added to the food. I started making my own beans and salsas. Chips are much better today, because you can find really good ones that have whole grains in them. Remember that blue corn has 20% more protein and 8% less starch. Colorful food is usually healthier than the less-colorful variety.

I make my beans and rice ahead of time and then have them ready to put together when I am ready. This is a good dish to serve to vegetarian guests. I also like to put this together and take to work for lunch. Just don't forget to take a fork!

Ingredients:

2½–3 c. cooked black beans (recipe p. 208)
2½–3 c. cooked whole-grain brown rice (recipe p. 208)
1 head romaine lettuce
1 bunch cilantro, chopped
1 tomato, chopped
1 pack whole-grain, organic tortilla chips (about 1 cup per person)

Directions: You may want to combine these steps on each individual serving plate, so each serving has a beautiful complete presentation.

1. Have black beans and rice warm and ready, set aside.
2. Tear lettuce into small, bite-sized pieces and put in bowl.
3. Add rice on top of lettuce. *(recipe continued on next page)*

4. Add black beans.
5. Sprinkle cilantro and tomato on top.
6. Crumble tortilla chips over top (about 1 cup per person).

Notes:

1. Use warm rice and beans warm.
2. Add sensational sea salt to taste. (see resources p. 299).

TEXAS CORNDOGS

I grew up eating corn dogs at the Texas State Fair. When I became a vegetarian, I missed them so much I decided to make my own. These were delicious and became one of my children's favorite meals! I don't add a stick to this corndog, but it tastes really great, anyway!

This recipe calls for tiny loaf pans that are made for baking bread. They are sold separately or as a large pan with individual, mini-loaf spaces. Many stores, including Sur La Table, Williams-Sonoma, Crate and Barrel, and Target, sell the pans. If you don't want to buy one, simply use a small cooking container that is about an inch and a half deep and longer than it is wide. This recipe will make about 12 mini corndogs.

Blue corn has 20% more protein and about 8% less starch than yellow cornmeal, though it does make your bread blue. Be sure to buy certified organic cornmeal. This recipe is fairly quick and easy, and, because it calls for quinoa flour, it is gluten-free.

Serve these warm with a little mustard or ketchup on the side.

Ingredients:

2 T. extra-virgin, pure coconut oil
1 c. whole cornmeal
½ c. quinoa flour
1½ T. baking powder (non-aluminum)
½ tsp. baking soda
½ tsp. sea salt
2 eggs
1½ c. buttermilk
2 T. ghee, melted
2 T. honey
1 pack vegetarian hot dogs

Directions:

1. Preheat oven to 450 degrees.
2. Place coconut oil in the tiniest loaf pans you can find, and let it melt in the oven for a couple of minutes. Remove from oven and set aside.
3. Sift together cornmeal, quinoa flour, baking powder, baking soda, and sea salt.

4. In a large bowl, beat eggs.
5. Add buttermilk, melted ghee, honey, and melted coconut oil to beaten eggs, and beat together.
6. Place a tiny piece of parchment paper in the bottom of each pan. Coat with coconut oil, and then turn it over and leave it in the bottom of the pan. (This will make it much easier to take out of the pan when it is finished.)
7. Cut hot dogs to fit into the pan lengthwise. Leave a little space at each end for the cornbread to cover it.
8. Add dry ingredients to wet ingredients.
9. Pour batter into the pans over parchment paper.
10. Place hot dogs in the center of the pan, so that they are surrounded by the corn bread on all sides.
11. Bake about 35 minutes. Tops should be golden brown and sides should have pulled away from the sides of the pan. (You can do the toothpick test to see if the center is done.)

Notes:

1. Have hot dogs ready. When the batter is ready, it is best to get it into the pans and then the oven very quickly.
2. Larger-sized hot dogs usually taste better.

VEGETARIAN MOO SHU

I loved moo shu pork when I used to eat meat. When I became a vegetarian, I started to make my own versions of foods I missed. This is a delicious, vegetarian version of moo shu.

Ingredients:

4–6 whole-grain tortillas
4 tsp. extra-virgin, pure coconut oil
4 eggs
¼ lb. mushrooms
4 c. cabbage, shredded
1 c. carrots, shredded
3 scallions, thinly sliced
2 T. teriyaki sauce
¼ c. raw peanuts, chopped
¼ c. hoisin sauce

Directions:

1. Preheat oven to 350 degrees.
2. Wrap tortillas in parchment paper and then wrap in foil, so that you don't have foil touching your food.

3. Heat tortillas in oven 5 to 8 minutes, just until they are warm.
4. Heat 2 tsp. of the coconut oil in a large skillet. Scramble three eggs, remove from skillet, and set aside.
5. Add remaining oil to skillet and sauté mushrooms until soft.
6. Add cabbage, carrots, scallions, and teriyaki sauce, and cook for another few minutes.
7. Beat remaining egg.
8. Add remaining egg to mixture and sauté a few moments.
9. Add peanuts and reserved eggs to the mixture and stir.
10. Take warm tortillas out of oven.
11. Taking one tortilla at a time, spread with a generous amount of hoisin sauce and then add a large spoonful of mushroom mixture.
12. Roll up tortillas.

Variation:

Substitute whole-grain pita bread for tortillas for more of a Middle Eastern version.

Side Dishes

BAKED SQUASH CASSEROLE

This recipe is really great in the fall or winter months. You can use yellow crook-necked squash or butternut squash.

Ingredients:

1½ T. extra-virgin, pure coconut oil
1 lb. squash, cut into chunks
¼ c. whole-grain quinoa flour
1 leek (white part only), chopped into small chunks
¾ c. cheddar cheese
1/8 tsp. nutmeg
1/8 tsp. ginger
½ tsp. sea salt
¼ tsp. pepper
1 c. cream or half-and-half

Directions:

1. Preheat oven to 350 degrees.
2. Grease a casserole dish with coconut oil.
3. Combine squash and flour, until squash is well-coated.
4. Place half of floured squash in the baking dish.
5. Put half of leeks in the baking dish, spreading them out evenly.
6. Sprinkle half of cheese over squash and leeks.
7. Add remaining squash and leeks evenly, over the cheese, and top with remaining cheese.
8. Mix nutmeg, ginger, sea salt, and pepper with cream.
9. Pour mixture evenly over all of squash, leeks, and cheese in the baking dish.
10. Bake 45–60 minutes.

Variation:

Use whatever whole-grain flour you desire. I use quinoa because it is complete protein , gluten-free and has a nice flavor. Whole-wheat works just as well.

BLACK-EYED PEAS

I grew up in Texas, where black-eyed peas and cornbread are a traditional meal. Leftovers of this meal freeze well.

Ingredients:

2 c. black-eyed peas
1 piece kombu seaweed
1 tsp. extra-virgin, pure coconut oil
½ c. onion, chopped
2 T. jalapeno, chopped
½ tsp. sea salt
¼ tsp. black pepper

Directions:

1. Soak black-eyed peas overnight in purified water.
2. Discard soaking water.
3. Put black-eyed peas in a large pot and add enough water to cover peas plus an additional inch. Bring to a boil.
4. Drain water.
5. Add enough new water to the pot to cover the peas by about an inch. Add seaweed, oil, onion, jalapeno, sea salt, and black pepper.
6. Bring to a boil, then reduce heat and simmer 30–45 minutes, or until the beans are soft.

Notes:

1. If you don't have time to soak black-eyed peas overnight, you will have to cook them a little longer.
2. Kombu seaweed can usually be found in the Asian foods area of Whole Foods Market, as well as other stores. Buy certified organic seaweed. Seaweed contributes many nutrients to any recipe and also helps break down the enzymes in beans and peas so they are more easily digested. You can discard it after cooking or eat it. I add it to almost all of my soups and beans when I am cooking them. There are a variety of seaweeds to choose from. They all have a variety of nutrients in them. Flavors vary. Experiment!

Variation:

For a little sweeter flavor, add a teaspoon of honey or maple syrup after this is removed from heat.

BROILED TOMATOES

I love tomatoes. This is one of those dishes I absolutely love on its own or with other dishes. It is great for breakfast, lunch, or dinner. If you have guests over and need a nice, quick side dish, this is a delicious choice. It also looks really beautiful on a formal dinner platter or plate.

Each tomato will serve one person. Serve warm.

Ingredients:

1 large tomato
sea salt to taste
pepper to taste
1 slice Parmesan (about ¼-inch thick; optional)

Directions:

1. Slice about ¼ inch off the top of tomato and cut out stem. You may need to slice a tiny bit off the bottom of the tomato to make it able to sit in the dish without falling over.
2. Season with salt and pepper to taste
3. Place cheese on top of tomato, if using.
4. Place tomato in a baking dish.
5. Broil (or bake at 350 degrees) until warm or until cheese is melted (about 8–10 minutes).

Variation:

Substitute cheddar or mozzarella for Parmesan.

BRUSSELS SPROUTS WITH CHESTNUTS

Chestnuts are low in fat, and high in protein and fiber. Here is an old, popular recipe served at many European holiday meals. It combines chewy chestnuts and Brussels sprouts for a wonderful taste.

Brussels sprouts are packed with vitamins and fiber, and are only about 25 calories per half-cup. Being a member of the disease-fighting cabbage family, they are also rich in phytochemicals that may protect us from cancer. Enjoy this delicious, healthy, and hearty dish any time, but it is especially good during the cold fall and winter months. This recipe makes enough for four to six people to enjoy.

Ingredients:

1 c. chestnuts
4 c. Brussels sprouts
2 T. extra-virgin, pure coconut oil
1 shallot, finely chopped
6 c. vegetable broth
1 T. butter
sea salt to taste
pepper to taste

Directions to cook chestnuts:

1. Using a small sharp knife, cut a cross at the bottom of each chestnut.
2. In a saucepan, bring 3 cups water to a boil. Gently drop in chestnuts using a slotted spoon, and boil about 8 minutes. (Use enough water to cover all of the chestnuts generously.)

3. Remove pan from heat and remove nuts a few at a time using a slotted spoon.
4. Gently remove the outer skin with a knife and peel off the inner skin.
5. Empty saucepan, put nuts and enough vegetable broth to just cover nuts, and put pan back on the heat.
6. Simmer about 15 minutes.
7. Drain nuts and set aside.

Directions:

1. Rinse and remove a few of the outer leaves of Brussels sprouts that might be yellow or wilted. (You can cut off the root end carefully to leave Brussels sprouts intact.)
2. In a heavy frying pan that has a lid, melt coconut oil and add shallot. Sauté for a few minutes, until shallot is soft.
3. Add Brussels sprouts and enough vegetable broth to just cover the sprouts. Cover and simmer on medium heat, stirring occasionally, about 8 minutes.
4. Add chestnuts, stir, cover, and cook until Brussels sprouts and chestnuts are tender, about 5 minutes.
5. Stir in butter, salt, and pepper.

COOKED BEANS

Beans are high in fiber, protein, and flavor. They are inexpensive and easy to store. Store uncooked, raw beans in a dark, cool, dry place. Beans are easy to freeze and thaw, so make a large batch and freeze some to use later. Beans are easy to add to salads or have as a side dish with soup or bread. Note that 1 pound of dried beans will yield about 5–6 cups cooked beans.

The optional seaweed in this recipe adds nutrients and helps make beans more digestible.

Ingredients:

1 lb. dried beans (any variety)
10 c. water, plus more for soaking and cooking
2-inch piece seaweed (optional)
sea salt to taste

Directions:

1. Check beans, and discard any that are shriveled or discolored.

Also check to make sure there are no little stones or foreign matter mixed in with beans.

2. Soak beans overnight in water. Make sure the dish is large enough for beans to double in size and enough water to cover them by at least 2 inches.
3. Pour off water.
4. In a 5-quart saucepan, bring 10 cups water and beans to a boil.
5. Discard water and keep beans.
6. Refill pot with new, purified water to about 2 inches over the top of beans. Add salt and seaweed, if using.
7. Bring water with beans to a boil again.
8. Reduce heat to a simmer, and cook beans until tender (about 45 minutes to an hour, depending on the size of beans; larger beans will take longer). Add more water if it gets too low and tops of beans are showing.
9. Remove from heat and they are ready to eat!

Variation:

Add a little bit of extra-virgin, pure coconut oil for extra richness.

NORI ROLLS WITH RICE

These easy, healthy, and delicious rolls really feed your body on a deep cellular level. Seaweed is a great way to add more iodine to the diet in a whole-food form. Nori kelp can be purchased in the Asian or ethnic foods section of the grocery store. It comes in sheets. The ingredients listed here make one roll.

Ingredients:

- nori sheet
- umeboshi paste
- sesame seeds
- whole-grain rice, cooked
- 1 avocado, cut into 1/2-inch-thick slices
- sea salt
- carrots, julienned
- cucumber, julienned
- sunflower or broccoli sprouts
- cilantro, chopped
- Nama Shoyu (unpasteurized raw soy sauce)
- wasabi (optional)
- pickled ginger (optional)

Directions:

1. Lay out nori sheet (shiny side down) on a flat surface or a bamboo (sushi) mat.

2. Spread a thin layer of umeboshi paste on a middle section of the nori sheet all the way across, about an inch high, leaving about a half inch border from the outside edge.
3. Sprinkle sesame seeds across the paste.
4. Spread rice in a thin layer over sesame seeds and paste, using your fingers. (Wet your fingers to make this easier.)
5. Spread avocado over rice, staying inside the edge about one-half inch.
6. Sprinkle avocado with a little sea salt.
7. Lay carrots and cucumbers in small amounts over avocado.
8. Sprinkle with sprouts and cilantro.
9. Take the end of the nori sheet right in front of you and start rolling it away from you.
10. Seal the edge with a little water.
11. Slice, using a sharp knife, into 1-inch-thick rolls.
12. Serve with soy sauce for dipping and wasabi and/or pickled ginger, if using.

Variation:

Mix a tiny bit of maple syrup or honey with the soy sauce to make it a little sweeter.

NUTTY SWEET RICE WITH LENTILS

Coconut oil, ghee, sea salt, and a vegetable bouillon cube add richness and flavor to this basic rice/lentil dish. If the bouillon cube you are using has salt in it, omit the salt in the recipe. As written, this recipe will serve six.

Ingredients:

- 2 c. whole-grain medium brown rice
- ¼ c. lentils
- ¼ tsp. sea salt
- 6 c. water
- 1–2 vegetable bouillon cubes, dissolved in the water
- 1 T. extra-virgin, pure coconut oil
- ½ c. pecans or walnuts, finely chopped
- ½ c. raisins
- 1 T. ghee (optional)
- ¼ c. raw coconut flakes

Directions:

1. Rinse rice and lentils in a small-weave sieve until they run clean.
2. Put rice, lentils, sea salt, water (with the bouillon cube dissolved in it), coconut oil, and half each of nuts and raisins in a large pot.
3. Bring to a boil; reduce heat to a simmer.
4. Cover the pot and do not disturb for 35–40 minutes. Do not stir.
5. When it looks as if all the water is absorbed, rice and lentils are ready.
6. Add ghee, if using, to rice and lentil mixture and gently toss.
7. Gently scoop out rice and lentils, and add coconut and remaining nuts and raisins.

Variation:

Add a little sautéed onion after cooking for a richer flavor.

QUINOA WITH BROCCOLI

Quinoa is gluten-free and is a complete protein. It is a nice alternative to rice. The darker variety has more anti-oxidants in it.

Ingredients:

2 c. quinoa
1 scallion, chopped
4 c. water
½ c. broccoli crowns, cut into bite-sized pieces
1/4 c. slivered almonds
2 T. olive oil
pinch of sea salt to taste

Directions:

1. Cook quinoa and all of the white part of the chopped scallion in water in a pot over a medium heat 15 to 20 minutes, until quinoa is soft. Remove from heat.
2. Add broccoli, almonds, remaining scallion, olive oil, and sea salt, and toss gently for a few moments until broccoli is a brighter green.

Notes:

1. Steam broccoli if you want softer broccoli.
2. I add broccoli after quinoa is already cooked and removed from heat in order to help retain more of the broccoli's nutritional value and live enzymes.

Variations:

1. Substitute ghee or extra-virgin, pure coconut oil for olive oil.
2. Add ¼ tsp. white truffle oil for more flavor.

ROASTED POTATOES WITH ROSEMARY

Potatoes and rosemary go really well together. I grow rosemary in my garden and love to add it to my dishes. This is a really easy recipe with a rich flavor that tastes comforting on a cold day. Note that new potatoes and red potatoes are the same.

Ingredients:

- 4 purple, Yukon gold, or red potatoes, cut in 2-inch chunks
- 3 T. sweet red onion, finely chopped
- 3 cloves garlic, freshly minced
- 2 T. rosemary
- 3 T. extra-virgin, pure coconut oil, slightly melted
- sea salt to taste
- pepper to taste
- 1 T. extra-virgin olive oil

Directions:

1. Preheat oven to 350 degrees.
2. Combine potatoes, onion, garlic, rosemary, coconut oil, salt, and pepper in a large baking dish. Make sure potatoes are well coated.
3. Bake 30 minutes, stir, and bake another 30 minutes.
4. Remove potatoes from oven, place in another dish, and toss with olive oil.

Notes:

1. You can melt coconut oil in the pan while it is preheating. This will make the oil easier to mix with the other ingredients. It will also coat the baking pan well.
2. To chop rosemary, remove leaves from stem and then chop leaves.

SAUTÉED ASPARAGUS

I love fresh vegetables. Though I eat asparagus raw a good deal of the time, this lightly sautéed dish is delicious. I love the combination of almonds and asparagus.

Serve this dish warm.

Ingredients:

2 lb. asparagus
1 T. extra-virgin, pure coconut oil
1 T. olive oil
sea salt to taste
pepper to taste
½ c. slivered almonds
½ c. Parmesan cheese (optional)

Directions:

1. Rinse asparagus and trim off thick, harder ends. Cut asparagus into approximately 2-inch pieces.
2. Sauté asparagus and coconut oil in a skillet or wok about 5 minutes over medium heat, until it becomes bright green and is just warm.
3. Drizzle olive oil over it and sprinkle with salt and pepper.
4. Sprinkle slivered almonds and Parmesan cheese, if using, on top.

Variation:

Use a mayonnaise and lemon juice sauce instead of olive oil.

STUFFED RED BELL PEPPERS

For this recipe, you need a lidded, deep baking dish that can hold bell peppers standing up straight. These are really delicious and nice to serve at dinner parties as a main dish. You can make them ahead of time and have them ready to bake. Serve them warm.

Each bell pepper will serve one person. Adjust the recipe accordingly.

Ingredients:

4 red bell peppers, seeds and stems removed, cleaned and halved
sea salt to taste
3 T. extra-virgin, pure coconut oil
1 sweet onion, finely chopped
2 celery stalks, finely chopped
2 carrots, finely chopped
4 c. quinoa, cooked
¼ c. fresh cilantro (or 1 T. dried)
2 T. fresh parsley, chopped
3 T. lemon juice

Directions:

1. Preheat oven to 375 degrees.
2. Cut off the bottom of each bell pepper very slightly, if you need to, so that peppers will sit on a flat surface. Sprinkle peppers lightly with sea salt and set aside.

3. Heat oil in large skillet over medium heat. Add onion, celery, and carrot.
4. Cover and cook until vegetables are softened (approximately 5 minutes), stirring as needed.
5. Add quinoa, cilantro, parsley, lemon juice, and sea salt, and stir to mix well. Taste and adjust seasonings if needed.
6. Stuff mixture into peppers.
7. Stand peppers up in baking dish, and pour ¼ inch water around (not over) peppers. Cover baking dish with lid.
8. Cook approximately 40–50 min or until peppers are fork-tender.

Note:

Try to buy peppers that will sit firmly on a flat surface.

Variation:

Substitute millet or rice for quinoa.

STUFFED TOMATOES

Each tomato will serve one person. Adjust the recipe accordingly for the number of people you are serving. The tomatoes are easy to save as leftovers. Simply refrigerate them, and warm them up later.

Ingredients:

8 medium tomatoes, halved lengthwise
¼ tsp. sea salt
1 c. parsley (fresh)
½ c. oregano (fresh)
1½ c. Parmesan cheese, finely grated
½ c. whole-grain bread crumbs
2 garlic cloves
1 shallot
2 T. extra-virgin olive oil

Directions:

1. Preheat oven to 400 degrees.
2. Core tomatoes and scoop out seeds. Reserve tomato insides.
3. Sprinkle 1/8 tsp. of the salt over the inside of tomatoes. Set aside.
4. In a food processor, combine parsley, oregano, Parmesan, bread crumbs, garlic, shallot, olive oil, and remaining sea salt. Pulse until herbs are chopped.

5. Chop the core of the tomato you removed, minus seeds and stems, and mix into herb mixture.
6. Pack filling into tomatoes, stuffing them to the top.
7. Place tomatoes, filling side up, on a baking dish and bake until shriveled and cheese is melted, about 12–15 minutes.
8. Remove from heat and let stand at least 5 minutes before serving.

Variation:

For more protein, add 1 cup cooked quinoa to filling before baking.

SWEET POTATO FRIES

I make sweet potato fries as a nutritious and easy snack in the afternoon (perfect for children right out of school) or as a side dish. I love easy baking recipes, because they can cook while I am busy doing other things. This dish really satisfies sweet and salty cravings.

You can have children rub the oil and sea salt on the potatoes. I find that children will eat a wider variety of healthy food if you involve them in the preparation process. Tell them they are chefs or scientific researchers! My daughter likes to make these super thin, in order for them to become crispier.

Ingredients:

2–3 sweet potatoes, washed well
2 T. extra-virgin, pure coconut oil
1–2 tsp. sea salt

Directions:

1. Preheat oven to 400 degrees.
2. Slice potatoes thinly (about ¼ of an inch thick) or slice into wedges. The thinner the wedge, the crispier it will get and the quicker it will cook.
3. Rub with coconut oil and sprinkle with sea salt.
4. Lay slices or wedges out on a large, flat, coconut oiled baking dish with low sides.
5. Bake until they are soft enough to put a fork into easily. (The time will depend on the thickness of the slices, maybe 25 to 40 minutes.)

6. After they are baked, place under the broiler for another 4 minutes or so in order to get them a little browner and crispier. Taste-test them carefully; you can judge how long it takes with your oven.

Notes:

These are best fresh, so only make as many as you are going to eat right away. Adjust the recipe accordingly.

SWEET POTATOES WITH CRANBERRIES AND APPLES

The sweet potato is sweet, but not the high-calorie indulgence most people think. It is actually about the same as a regular white potato. It has about 105 calories per 3½ ounces. It is actually not even a potato; it is of the morning glory family. It is packed with Vitamin A and beta carotene. This high-fiber food is a wonderful way to add color and variety to a meal. This recipe is a nutritious and colorful side dish. It also makes a nice holiday side dish. It is a beautiful blend of sweet and tart flavors. This recipe makes eight servings.

Ingredients:

5 sweet potatoes, peeled and cut in 1-inch chunks
2 T. butter
1 large green apple, cored, peeled, and diced
1 c. raw cranberries
½ c. raisins
1 T. honey or raw sugar
½ c. orange juice

Directions:

1. Preheat oven to 350 degrees F.
2. Place sweet potatoes in a large, buttered baking dish, and top with apples, cranberries, and raisins.
3. Drizzle with honey or raw sugar.
4. Pour orange juice over top.
5. Cover and bake for 1 hour and 15 minutes, or until sweet potatoes are tender when pierced with a fork.

Variation:

Substitute yams for sweet potatoes.

Variations:

1. Add ¼ cup chopped pecans or walnuts.
2. Substitute dried cranberries for fresh.

SWISS CHARD WITH SAUTÉED MUSHROOMS

I love to make this recipe whenever I have Swiss chard fresh from my garden. It makes a great side dish, or a quick and easy vegetarian main dish. Shitake mushrooms are a great choice for this recipe, but you can use any variety. Depending on portion sizes, it will serve four to six people.

Ingredients:

1 bunch Swiss chard, washed
1 T. extra-virgin, pure coconut oil
1 T. ghee or butter
¼ c. red onion, chopped
2 c. mushrooms, brushed, rinsed, and sliced
3 T. warm water
1 T. miso
1 tsp. garlic, minced
sea salt to taste
pepper to taste

Directions:

1. Stack Swiss chard leaves, roll up, and cut crossways into strips.
2. Set Swiss chard aside.
3. Melt coconut oil and ghee or butter in a large skillet over medium heat. Add onion and sauté 1–2 minutes.
4. Add mushrooms and sauté until onion gets a little clear and soft, about 3–4 minutes.
5. Mix warm water and miso until miso makes a kind of broth.
6. Add miso broth to skillet and incorporate.
7. Add Swiss chard to skillet and sauté lightly until it is bright green and wilts. (This takes only a few minutes.)
8. Add garlic, salt, and pepper, and sauté lightly for a few seconds.
9. Remove from heat.

Notes:

1. Add a little more onion if you love onions.
2. Add a little more water or oil if onions seem to get too dry while you're sautéing them.

Variation:

Garnish with fresh chopped parsley.

TOM SPICER'S BROWN RICE AND CHESTNUTS

My friend Tom Spicer owns Farm Road 1410, a produce company in Dallas, Texas, that provides amazing fresh, mostly organic food of all varieties. He is the fresh produce provider for most of the top gourmet chefs in town. He gave me another recipe for this book (Tahini Dip for Tom Spicer's Steamed Vegetables with Tahini Dip; recipe on page 231), and he suggests putting the recipes together for a complete meal. He made this for our dinner one night and it was absolutely scrumptious.

Ingredients:

2 c. whole long-grain rice
5 c. water
1- to 2-inch-piece kombu seaweed
¾–1 c. chestnuts, peeled
sea salt to taste

Directions:

1. Rinse rice until it runs clear.
2. Place rice, water, kombu seaweed, and chestnuts into a large pot.
3. Bring rice to a boil and stir for a few moments.
4. Reduce heat to low, cover with a tight-fitting lid, and simmer without stirring about 40 minutes.
5. Fluff rice with a fork and leave it in the pot, off of heat, about 5 to 10 minutes. (This will give you drier, fluffier rice.)
6. Sea salt to taste

Note:

While it is still warm, you can also place the rice chestnut mixture in a wood bowl, cover with a warm dish towel, and let sit a few minutes.

WHOLE-GRAIN RICE WITH BOUILLON

Coconut oil, ghee, sea salt, and bouillon cube add more richness and flavor to a basic rice dish. If the bouillon cube you are using has salt in it, do not add additional salt. This recipe yields approximately six servings.

Ingredients:

2 c. whole-grain brown basmati rice
6 c. water
¼ tsp. sea salt (optional)
1 T. extra-virgin, pure coconut oil (optional)
1–2 vegetable bouillon cubes, dissolved in the water
1–2 T. ghee (optional)

Directions:

1. Rinse rice thoroughly in a small-weave sieve until water runs clear. Set aside.
2. Bring water to a boil in a large pot. Add rice, sea salt, if using, coconut oil, if using, and bouillon cube(s), and let boil for a couple of minutes while stirring.
3. Reduce heat to a simmer.
4. Cover pot tightly and do not disturb for 35 to 40 minutes. Do not stir.
5. When it looks as if all the water is absorbed, rice is ready.
6. Let rice sit in the pot off of the heat about 5 minutes. Fluff rice with a fork.
7. Add ghee, if using, and stir gently.
8. Gently scoop out the rice and serve warm.

Note:

Long-grain rice is fluffier, whereas medium-grain is a little moister.

Variations:

1. Add a little sautéed onion to this after cooking for a richer and different flavor.
2. Add some raisins and pine nuts for a different sweet and nutty flavor.
3. Substitute whole-grain quinoa for rice. (It will cook in about half the time.)

Spreads, Dips, and Dressings

Raw recipe

CREAMY AVOCADO DRESSING

This is one of my favorite dressings. Serve it over salad greens or sprouts with some sunflower seeds, or use it as a sandwich spread.

Ingredients:

- 1 avocado
- 2–3 T. fresh lemon juice
- 1 clove garlic, freshly minced
- 1 T. honey
- 1 pinch sea salt
- 3 T. extra-virgin olive oil

Directions:

1. Combine avocado, lemon juice, garlic, honey, and sea salt.
2. Add olive oil in a slow, steady stream while blending the other ingredients.

Variation:

1. Substitute balsamic vinegar for lemon juice.
2. Substitute 1 cup chopped cucumber for honey.

GARLIC SALT BUTTER

My mother taught me to make this spread when we were having Italian food. The healthful benefits of the garlic and sea salt give it an added bonus!

Ingredients:

- ½ c. ghee or butter (unsalted), softened
- 1 T. parsley (fresh or dried), chopped
- 1 or 2 cloves garlic, minced
- 1/8 tsp. sea salt

Directions:

1. Combine all ingredients by hand with a fork or with a food processor.

Notes:

1. For an easier, quicker version, simply mix butter and and store-bought garlic salt.
2. Use right away or store in a tightly sealed container in the refrigerator.

HERB BUTTER

I love rich herb butter on my bread when I am having soup or an Italian dish. This is a slight variation of my Garlic Salt Butter (recipe on page 223). I serve this for people who are sensitive to garlic; it is always nice to give people a choice. I usually spread it on big, thick slices of crusty, whole-grain bread, wrap it up, warm up the loaf, and serve it warm. Yum! It also makes a very nice spread for little finger sandwiches to serve with tea in the afternoon.

If you aren't using right away, store this in a tightly sealed container in the refrigerator.

Ingredients:

½ c. ghee (room temperature)
2 T. parsley (fresh or dried), finely chopped
½ tsp. thyme (fresh or dried), finely chopped

Directions:

1. Combine all ingredients by hand with a fork or in a food processor.

HUMMUS

Hummus is a Mediterranean dip that is delicious and so easy to make. It is high in protein, mostly raw and uncooked, and easy to eat. I have played with making so many hummus recipes that I now call myself the hummus queen! I use different oils, different beans, and different butters.

Serve on whole-grain pita bread, crackers, or bread, or with fresh vegetables slices.

Ingredients:

1 c. white northern beans, pinto beans, or chickpeas (cooked)
¼ c. lemon juice (fresh)
1 clove garlic, minced
1½ T. raw tahini
1 T. raw cashew butter
1 tsp. cumin
¼ c. parsley (fresh)
3 T. extra-virgin olive oil
¼–½ tsp. sea salt (to taste)

Directions:

1. Combine all ingredients in food processor and mix well.

Variations:

1. Add ¼ teaspoon black or white pepper.
2. Add 1 tablespoon macadamia nut oil.

MINT YOGURT

This dish is a Middle Eastern Favorite known as tzatziki. It is cool and refreshing on hot summer days. It can be eaten as a soup, as a dip, or with breads, vegetables, or fresh fruit. Serve it chilled. As written, this recipe serves four.

Ingredients:

2 c. plain yogurt
1 cucumber, peeled, seeded, and grated
1 tsp. fresh mint leaves (finely chopped)
1 scallion, peeled and finely chopped
1 T. fresh lemon juice
½ tsp. Sensational Sea Salt
pepper to taste

Directions:

1. Place all ingredients in a bowl and blend well.
2. Chill in the refrigerator for at least an hour before serving.
3. Serve

Notes:

1. Coconut yogurt works well in this recipe.
2. It is best nutritionally to eat this immediately after blending.
3. Sensational Sea Salt is listed in the Resources. It is Nancy's patent pending salt blend that supports the thyroid.

Variations:

1. Use the whole cucumber and leave the peel on cucumber for its nutritional benefits and blend the recipe in a food processor or blender, instead of by hand, but blending it will make it more like a soup.
2. Substitute dill for mint.

Raw recipe

MOCK HOLLANDAISE SAUCE

Mom always served this with cooked artichokes or asparagus. It was one of Papa's favorite dishes. Serve this with steamed vegetables like artichokes, broccoli, and cauliflower.

Ingredients:

3 T. butter
2 T. whole-grain flour
½ tsp. sea salt
2/3 c. milk or goat milk
2 T. lemon juice
2 egg yolks, well beaten

Directions:

1. Melt butter in a saucepan, and then blend in flour and sea salt.
2. Add milk and cook, stirring constantly, over direct heat until sauce boils and thickens.
3. Remove from heat.
4. Add lemon juice.
5. Place egg yolks in a double-boiler.
6. Stir butter mixture into egg yolks.
7. Place double boiler over boiling water and cook, stirring constantly, 2 minutes, until sauce is smooth and thick.

Note:

Whole-wheat pastry flour works well in this recipe, but you can use oat or quinoa flour for a non-gluten flour.

Raw recipe

OLIVE OIL AND BALSAMIC VINEGAR DIPPING SAUCE

This is delicious served with crusty whole-grain bread or whole grain focaccia bread. It pairs well with Italian or Greek food.

Serve this in individual dipping bowls with bread.

Ingredients:

½ c. extra-virgin olive oil
2½ T. balsamic vinegar
1 T. freshly ground black pepper

Directions:

1. Stir ingredients together.

Raw recipe

PESTO

This is one of my favorite ways to use fresh basil from my garden. It is so versatile. I use this pesto for so many dishes: as a pasta sauce, to stuff mushrooms, to spread on tomatoes, as a salad dressing, on pizza, as a topping for bread—the possibilities are endless!

Keep the olive oil sealing the top. Every time you use it, if you seal it back up, it will keep for a long, long time. Just clean up the sides of the jar and seal it up with olive oil.

Ingredients:

1¾ c. pine nuts
2 c. basil
¼ c. walnuts
1/3 c. extra-virgin olive oil
½ tsp. sea salt.
½ tsp. black pepper

Directions:

1. Combine all ingredients in food processor and process until smooth.
2. Place in a jar with a good-fitting lid. Make sure the inside of the jar is cleaned of food, all the way down to the top of mixture.
3. Cover top of mixture with at least ¼ inch of olive oil.

Notes:

1. Store in refrigerator.
2. Soak nuts 12 to 18 hours and then dehydrate them on low, if you wish to remove some of the phytic acid.

Variation:

Add ¼ c. Parmesan cheese.

Raw recipe

PICO DE GALLO

Pico de gallo is a healthy and delicious condiment commonly served with Mexican food. It goes well with bean dishes, egg dishes, guacamole, and tortilla chips. Pico de gallo is easy to make, and you can keep it in the refrigerator for a few days in a well-sealed container.

Ingredients:

8 tomatoes, diced
1 onion, diced
1/3 c. cilantro, chopped
2 (or more) jalapeños, seeded and minced
sea salt to taste

Directions:

1. Combine all ingredients in a bowl.
2. Place in refrigerator for an hour or overnight to allow flavors to meld together.

Variation:

Substitute chilis or milder peppers, like Serrano or chipotle, for jalapeños.

POPPY SEED DRESSING

This dressing can be refrigerated for up to a week.

Ingredients:

2 T. lemon juice
2 T. apple cider vinegar
3 T. maple syrup
2 T. poppy seeds
pinch of sea salt
2 T. sunflower, safflower, walnut, or or extra-virgin olive oil
2/3 c. plain yogurt

Directons:

1. Mix lemon juice, vinegar, maple syrup, poppy seeds, and sea salt together until maple syrup is dissolved well.
2. Stir in oil and yogurt.

Variation:

Substitute honey for maple syrup.

PUMPKIN BUTTER

Serve this with breads, pancakes, or waffles.

Ingredients:

1 c. ghee or butter, softened
½ c. pumpkin puree
1 pinch sea salt
½ tsp. maple syrup or honey

Directions:

1. Place all ingredients in food processor and blend until pureed and creamy.

HOW TO COOK A PUMPKIN

Cut pumpkin in two. Take a large spoon and scrape out insides of the pumpkin. (If you want to save the seeds to plant in your garden or make roasted pumpkin seeds, put them aside on a tray or plate to dry.)

Take the two halves of the pumpkin and place them open-side down on a large baking pan. Bake at 350 degrees until pumpkin is soft.

Remove from oven and let cool. When cool, place in a food processor and blend with the large blade until it's a creamy puree.

You can use this in recipes or freeze it for future use.

Raw recipe

SALSA

Here in Texas, we use salsa as a side dish for many of our meals. This is a very basic, easy recipe.

Ingredients:

6 tomatoes
2 jalapeño peppers, de-stemmed
4 T. fresh cilantro (optional)

Directions:

1. Place all ingredients in blender and blend well.

Variation:

Increase jalapeños for a hotter flavor.

Raw recipe

SALSA (WITH A KICK!)

Chef Paco Carenas in San Miguel de Allende, Mexico, gave me this recipe. Use really fresh ingredients. You can probably find some of the ingredients in a Mexican grocery store. Serve this with tortilla chips.

Ingredients:

8 pieces prickly pear (Xoconostles)
4 chile mora
2 garlic cloves, peeled
1/3 medium onion
sea salt to taste

Directions:

1. Roast all ingredients in a dry skillet over medium heat.
2. When chiles are soft, place them in a small saucepan with boiling water for about 10 minutes.
3. In the meantime, peel each prickly pear, cut in half, discard inside seeds, cut in small pieces, and set aside.
4. Put chiles, roasted garlic, and some salt in a molcajete (Mexican volcanic rock mortar and pestle) and mash to a puree. (This can also be done in a food processor.)
5. Add roasted onion and continue to smash really well.
6. Add chopped prickly pear, mix together, and sprinkle with additional sea salt to taste.

Raw recipe

SWEET AND SOUR SAUCE

I love sweet and sour sauce. I tried to find one at the supermarket that didn't have a lot of additives in it, gave up, and invented this one. The dates give it a little body as well as sweetness. If you like it very sweet, add a couple more dates to the recipe. This recipe has sweet, sour, and salty flavors, so it can really satisfy some cravings. Use this as a dipping sauce for egg rolls, cooked tofu, meats, or freshly cut vegetables like tomatoes.

This recipe makes one serving. You can double or triple this recipe, and keep in the refrigerator for up to one week.

Ingredients:

4 T. apple cider vinegar
3 T. extra-virgin olive oil
3-4 dates soaked in water (for about an hour)
½ tsp. soy sauce (raw and organic)

Directions:

1. Place all ingredients in blender and blend.

Variation:

Substitute balsamic vinegar for apple cider vinegar.

TAHINI DIP for Tom Spicer's Steamed Vegetables with Tahini Dip

Tom is an amazing organic gardener who owns Farm Road 1410 in Dallas. He provides many of gourmet restaurant chefs, as well as many other clients, with exotic and fresh produce. He is a celebrity in the Dallas–Ft. Worth area in the area of top-quality organics. He is a gourmet chef himself, as well as having some amazing chefs working at his garden establishment.

He serves this dish with his Tom Spicer's Brown Rice and Chestnuts (recipe on page 218) for a wonderful, full-flavored meal. This can be a side dish, a main dish, or a snack/appetizer.

I love to serve this dip with steamed vegetables for any type of party I have in the fall or winter. It is absolutely delicious!

Steamed Vegetables Ingredients:

1 c. daikon radish
1 c. parsnips
1 c. carrots
1 c. broccoli
1 c. snow peas

Dip Ingredients:

1 block organic tofu (medium soft)
2–3 T. Italian parsley
2 scallions, finely chopped
1 T. dark miso
1 T. umeboshi paste
1 c. raw tahini butter
1 T. tamari
1 T. lemon juice
½ c. golden toasted sesame seeds*
1 T. ginger juice (freshly grated and squeezed to produce the juice)
sea salt to taste

Directions:

1. Slice tofu lengthwise into four layers. Place each layer on a cotton dish towel and wrap it up. Place a cutting board or something with weight on top of it. (This will help drain most of the moisture out of the tofu.)
2. Chop parsley and set aside.
3. Chop scallions and set aside.
4. Mash tofu into a thick, mushy consistency.
5. Combine tofu, miso, umeboshi paste, tahini butter, tamari, and lemon juice in a bowl. Use a potato masher or a large fork to mash really well.
6. Add half each of parsley, scallions, and sesame seeds to tofu mixture. Combine by hand and set aside.
7. Add ginger juice and salt to tofu mixture.
8. Cut radish, parsnips, and carrots in a thin diagonal.
9. Cut broccoli into bite-sized pieces.
10. Trim off ends of snow peas.
11. Place radish, parsnips, carrots, broccoli, and snow peas in a vegetable steamer and steam lightly.
12. Place dip in a bowl and top with the remaining parsley, scallions, and sesame seeds.

***To make golden toasted sesame seeds:** Put sesame seeds in a pan over low heat and stir until they start to pop. Take them off heat quickly. (They should be golden brown.) Sprinkle with a pinch of sea salt and set aside.

Note:

When you are trimming vegetables to use as pretty foods for dipping in the dip, save the ends and leftover vegetable pieces that you are not using in your recipe to make a vegetable broth, or add them when you make fresh vegetable juice.

Soups

ASPARAGUS-POTATO SOUP

This is one of my absolute favorite soups. A woman from India shared this recipe with me as we sat and watched our daughters practice gymnastics. I changed it just a little bit over the years. Everyone who eats it just loves it. Milk makes the soup richer and creamier. I leave the skins on the potatoes in this recipe.

Be careful when blending hot ingredients. The steam and heat can build up, and it can explode though the top of the blender, burning you and making a terrible mess. I always do it very carefully with small amounts, and I cover the blender with a large dish towel to help protect me (and the kitchen) from a mess.

Ingredients:

- 1 onion, chopped in large pieces
- 2 T. ghee, butter, or extra-virgin, pure coconut oil
- 1 bunch asparagus
- 3 large sweet potatoes
- 6 c. water
- 1 tsp. sea salt
- 1 c. milk (any variety)

Directions:

1. Sauté onion in ghee, butter, or oil in a large soup pot, until onion starts to look a little clear.
2. Cut off and discard hard ends of the asparagus (about a half inch).
3. Cut asparagus and potatoes in large chunks.
4. Add asparagus to onion mixture and sauté a moment more.
5. Add water, potatoes, and sea salt, and bring to a boil.
6. Reduce heat and cook over medium heat until potatoes are tender.
7. Remove from heat.
8. When soup is cooler, blend mixture in blender until creamy.
9. Add milk, if using.

Variation:

Use another type of potato. The original recipe called for russet potatoes, but any variety is delicious. I love the sweet potato flavor, and they have more color to them. Purple potatoes taste great, but look a little purple!

BLACK BEAN SOUP

This recipe is a very easy one that you can cook in a slow cooker. If you want a warm meal when you get home from work or being out all day, this rich and satisfying dish is a great choice. Serve it with whole-grain bread for a wonderful supper.

Ingredients:

- 1½ c. black beans
- 10–12 c. water
- 1 red onion, diced
- 3 stalks celery, chopped into half-inch chunks
- 3 carrots, chopped into bite-sized chunks
- 2 T. extra-virgin, pure coconut oil
- 2 vegetable bouillon cubes
- 1 c. hot water
- 3 garlic cloves, minced
- 1 tsp. sea salt
- ½ tsp. black pepper
- 1 tsp. turmeric
- 1 tsp. coriander
- 1 tsp. chili powder
- 2 tsp. savory

Directions:

1. Soak beans overnight in water.
2. Pour off water.
3. Sauté onion, celery, and carrots 5 minutes in oil.
4. Place in slow cooker.
5. Bring beans in a large pot (not the slow cooker) and about 4 cups of water (enough water to cover them by at least an inch) to a boil, and then drain off water.
6. In a small dish dissolve bouillon cubes in 1 cup hot water.
7. Place beans in slow cooker with remaining ingredients, including dissolved bouillon, 6 additional cups of water, and herbs and spices.
8. Turn on slow cooker and cook 6–8 hours on low.

Variations:

1. Serve with a big dollop of milk, rich crème, or sour cream.
2. Sprinkle with chopped parsley and chives as garnish.
3. Substitute oregano, parsley, and thyme for savory and coriander.

LENTIL SOUP

Serve this with crusty, whole-grain bread.

Ingredients:

2 T. extra-virgin, pure coconut oil
2 onions, chopped
3 carrots, chopped
¾ tsp. marjoram
¾ tsp. thyme
½ tsp. salt (or to taste)
¼ tsp. black pepper
3 c. tomatoes (crushed or diced)
7 c. water
1 c. lentils, rinsed
1/3 c. fresh or 2 T. dried parsley
½ c. or more grated cheddar cheese (optional)

Directions:

1. Sauté oil, onions, carrots, marjoram, thyme, salt, and pepper about 4–5 minutes in a large soup pot.
2. Add tomatoes and stir for a couple of minutes.
3. Add water and lentils.
4. Bring to a boil, then reduce heat to a simmer and cook 45 minutes, or until lentils are soft.
5. Remove from heat and add parsley.
6. Sprinkle with cheese, if using.
7. Serve warm.

MISO SOUP WITH MUSHROOMS

This is such an easy, delicious soup. I frequently make this to sip in the afternoon, instead of afternoon tea. It is a high-protein, nutrient-rich, and probiotic-rich soup.

Ingredients:

10 dried shitake mushrooms, sliced
4½ c. water
¼ c. miso
¼ c. chopped watercress for garnish (optional)

Directions:

1. Soak mushrooms at least 10 minutes in ½ cup water, until soft.
2. Simmer 4 cups water in a pan. Do not boil.
3. Add miso and stir until miso is dissolved.
4. Remove from heat.

5. Add mushrooms and their soaking liquid when miso water is just warm enough to drink.
6. Add chopped watercress, if using, as a garnish.

Variation:

Add kombu seaweed for additional nutrition.

NUTRITIOUS BROTH WITH MUSHROOMS AND GARLIC

One of my acupuncturists, Sunny, told me once to make a soup using zucchini, carrots, celery, potatoes (I like to use colored ones, like purple or sweet), and a sweet onion. I started making this broth and then started adding seaweed to it as well. I drain off the vegetables after I make it and drink the broth. You can save the vegetables and eat them, or eat it all together as a vegetable soup.

I add the garlic last, because it is fragile. Garlic has anticancer characteristics; it may lower breast, colon, stomach, throat, and skin cancer risks. It has both antibiotic and antifungal properties. The secret to its health benefits? Sulfides. The sulfides aren't released unless the garlic is crushed or chopped, and then left to sit at least 10 to 15 minutes before eating. Add more garlic if you want a more medicinal soup. Drink this while it is warm.

This recipe is very alkalizing as well.

Ingredients:

4 carrots, cut in small chunks
½ c. peas
1 zucchini, cut in small chunks
2 celery stalks, cut in small chunks
1–2 potatoes (preferably purple potatoes, yams, or sweet potatoes, not white potatoes), cut in small chunks
½ onion, cut in small chunks
2-inch-piece kombu seaweed
sea salt to taste (optional)
5 c. water
1 or 2 cloves garlic, finely minced
¼ c. mushrooms, sliced

Directions:

1. Place carrots, peas, zucchini, celery, potatoes, onion, seaweed, and sea salt in a large pot with water in it and bring to a boil.
2. Reduce heat and simmer about 20 minutes, until potatoes are tender.
3. Strain vegetables.
4. Add garlic and mushrooms.
5. Serve warm.

Salads

AMANDA'S INDIAN SALAD

My daughter, Amanda, loves to cook. When she got back from serving two years in Mali, West Africa, with the Peace Corps, she started inventing wonderful dishes. This is one of my favorites. As written, this makes one serving.

Ingredients:

1 c. mixed baby greens
1/3 c. chopped tomato
1 c. warm, cooked green lentils
1 tsp. minced red onion
1 T. extra-virgin olive oil
¼ tsp. curry powder
¼ tsp. turmeric
sea salt to taste
fresh ground pepper to taste

Directions:

1. Combine all ingredients well and enjoy!

APPLE SALAD

The apple is one of the most nutritious foods, with remedies dating back to the earliest times of history. One medium apple, fresh, raw, and with the skin, has high levels of Vitamin C, potassium, iron, calcium, phosphorus, Vitamin A, boron, and folate—and only 81 calories. In addition, the fiber content of one apple is equivalent to a serving of bran cereal.

This simple recipe is a variation of the Waldorf salad recipe I learned from my mother. This recipe makes a great light lunch to pack for school or work.

Salad Ingredients:

3 T. lemon juice
3 large red apples, cored and cut in bite-sized pieces
2/3 c. pineapple (preferably fresh), cut in bite-sized pieces
1/3 c. celery, diced
¼ c. raisins
¼ c. grapes
¼ c. pecan pieces

Recipe continued on next page

Dressing Ingredients:

3 T. plain yogurt
2 tsp. mayonnaise
1T. honey
¼ tsp. cinnamon

Directions:

1. In a bowl, mix lemon juice and apple pieces.
2. In a medium bowl, combine all salad ingredients.
3. In a small bowl, mix together dressing ingredients.
4. Mix dressing with salad ingredients.

Note:

Lemon juice will keep apple pieces from turning brown.

Variation:

Substitute walnuts for pecans.

Raw recipe

BROCCOLI AND SUNFLOWER SEED SALAD

When you make this salad, make it about an hour before you want to serve it so that the flavors can meld together before serving. Store it in the refrigerator. This salad is excellent as leftovers the next day. It is also makes a super salad for lunch on the go! This recipe makes a lot, so you can serve this at a dinner or save some for the next few days to have for lunch. Each cup of broccoli will serve about one person.

Salad Ingredients:

10 c. broccoli crowns
1 c. sunflower seeds
¼ c. pumpkin seeds
1 c. dates, chopped
¾ c. red onion, chopped finely

Dressing Ingredients:

1 c. milk of choice
1 avocado
4 T. apple cider vinegar
¾ tsp. sea salt
¼ c. extra-virgin olive oil
3 T. honey

Directions:

1. Combine all salad ingredients in a large bowl and set aside.
2. Combine all dressing ingredients in a blender and blend.
3. Combine dressing with salad ingredients in the large bowl, and toss well.

Variation:

Substitute raisins or currants for dates.

GRANNY'S CARROT RAISIN SALAD

I love this salad. It always reminds me of my childhood days spent at my grandmother's home. When I make this salad, I make a double recipe. I like to have it handy for easy snacks or a part of meals throughout the week. I leave the peel on the carrots, because they are full of nutrients.

Ingredients:

1 bag carrots, not peeled, grated
1–2 c. raisins
¼ c. mayonnaise

Directions:

1. Mix all ingredients together and enjoy!

Variation:

Substitute ¼ cup orange juice mixed with 2 tablespoons raw, organic, extra-virgin, pure coconut oil for mayonnaise.

MIDDLE EASTERN BEAN SALAD WITH PITA BREAD

I have heard many people say they just get tired of eating salads. This salad has flavor and is easy to prepare. This is a nice alternative to a basic garden salad and would make a great lunch to take to school or work.

Ingredients:

1½ c. cooked pinto, kidney, or black beans
3 scallions, chopped
½ c. diakon radish, finely chopped
1 c. cucumber, chopped
½ c. red bell pepper, chopped
1 clove garlic, minced
¼ c. lemon juice (fresh)
4 T. extra-virgin olive oil
4 T. pine nuts
1 T. sesame seeds
½ tsp. paprika
½ tsp. oregano
½ tsp. parsley
2 T. dill (fresh)
½ tsp. sea salt
whole-grain pita bread
4 c. romaine lettuce, chopped

Directions:

1. In a large bowl, combine beans, scallions, radish, cucumber, red bell pepper, garlic, lemon juice, olive oil, pine nuts, sesame seeds, paprika, oregano, parsley, dill, and sea salt. Let sit at least 15–20 minutes in order for the juices to meld together.

2. Warm pita bread in the oven for about 5 minutes, then drizzle with a touch of olive oil, and sprinkle with a pinch of sea salt, parsley, and oregano. Keep warm until serving.
3. Add lettuce to bean mixture and toss lightly.

Note:

1. Dried herbs work, but fresh herbs are really wonderful in this dish.
2. Only add lettuce right before you are going to serve the salad. If you are going to store any of this salad for taking as lunch later on, for example, don't add lettuce to the part you are going to save. The lettuce will wilt if it is stored in this way.

Variations:

1. Toast sesame seeds in a skillet for a toasty fragrant version.
2. Toast pita bread in the oven for a crispier pita. Cut into wedges.

Raw recipe

SPINACH SALAD

I used to make this for my children and their friends. This is one of my son's favorite salads. It's an easy salad recipe. I have found that many people who usually don't like salad enjoy this one.

Ingredients:

1 bunch spinach (fresh)
1 c. raw almond slivers
2 tangerines or oranges, peeled, seeded, and sectioned
½ c. sprouts
Poppy Seed Dressing (recipe on page 228)

Directions:

1. Tear spinach into bite-sized pieces.
2. Add almonds, tangerines or oranges, and sprouts.
3. Toss with dressing.
4. Top with more sprouts.

Variation:

Substite canned mandarin oranges for tangerines or oranges.

SUZIE HUMPHREYS'S GREEK SALAD

My friend Suzie makes the best Greek salad! She generously gave me the recipe for my book.

Ingredients:

1 c. romaine lettuce, torn in bite-sized pieces
1 cucumber, peeled, seeded, and chopped
1 red pepper, seeded and chopped
¼ c. red onion, cut into small, thin silvers
¼ c. black olives
¼ c. green onions
1 stalk celery, chopped
1 tomato, chopped
¾ c. feta cheese (raw, organic, and with vegetable enzymes)
La Martinique salad dressing

Directions:

1. Toss all ingredients together with salad dressing.

Variation:

Substitute another vinaigrette salad dressing for La Martinique dressing.

Breads

AUNT KATHERINE'S YEAST ROLLS

This is an old family recipe of Edna Ridley Gibbons. My mother learned this recipe from my Great-Aunt Katherine in the late 1950s. That is where it got its name. My mother makes these rolls for every special dinner and other occasion my family celebrates together. The nephews and nieces have begged for lessons on how to make this special and beloved recipe. My mother gives lessons to her grandchildren when she makes them for our Christmas breakfast or Thanksgiving dinner. She learned to make this recipe with white, refined flour and sugar; I have changed the recipe to use healthier ingredients. Our family likes to serve these rolls with butter or jam, or we make little sandwiches with them.

Note that oat and quinoa are gluten-free flours and will keep the bread from being as sticky as whole-wheat flour. (You can substitute ½ c. glutinous rice flour for ½ c. oat or quinoa flour for celiac-intolerant people and get a little bit of a stickier version.) Whole-grain flour is heavier, so you don't need as much flour as you would if you were using white, refined flour. I use about 6 cups total flour for this recipe. I use the remaining cup for sprinkling on the board when I roll out the dough to cut the rolls.

Ingredients:

2 T. dry yeast
2 c. lukewarm water
½ c. raw turbinado sugar or xylitol
1 egg, well beaten
1 tsp. sea salt
6–7 sifted c. whole-grain flour
3 T. + ½ c. extra-virgin, pure coconut oil, melted

Directions:

1. Put yeast in a large bowl and dissolve in lukewarm water, mixing well.
2. Add sugar and mix well.
3. Add egg, salt, and about 3 cups of the flour. Beat until smooth.
4. Add 3 T. melted coconut oil and mix well.
5. Add remaining flour, one cup at a time, and mix. (If dough is heavy and dense, you may want to only add 3 cups of the remaining flour), and then beat well.
6. Cover with wax paper and let rise for about two hours (preferably in a warm place) or until it has doubled in size.
7. Remove half of dough, knead a few minutes on a lightly floured board, and roll out on a floured board.

8. Cut with a biscuit cutter.
9. Dip biscuits into ½ cup warm, melted coconut oil, fold once, and place on a greased pan in a line next to each other. (They should form lines across.)
10. Repeat process with remaining dough.
11. Preheat oven to 425 degrees.
12. Let biscuits rise another hour.
13. Bake 6 to 10 minutes. (Do not overcook.)

Notes:

1. Sift flour before measuring.
2. Rolls can be made ahead of time (up to a week in advance). Rolls can be cooked lightly, and then left to cool to room temperature. Once rolls are room temperature, leave in the pan, and then wrap the whole pan and rolls really well and put them in the freezer. When you're ready to use, take out of the freezer and thaw (this can take anywhere from two to four hours), then warm up in the oven about 4–8 minutes. Watch them closely so they don't overcook.

Variation:

Bake this in loaf pans: Grease two loaf pans with coconut oil and put parchment paper in the bottom of the pans before putting dough into the pan to rise. After I make the bread dough, I let it rise in the bowl for about two hours. Next, knead dough lightly one more time on a lightly floured board. Then divide in half. Put half into each loaf pan (it should be about half full), and then let rise for another hour before baking in the loaf pan. Bake at 425 degrees 45 minutes to an hour, or until the top is toasty brown and the sides of the bread have pulled away from the sides of the pan.

AUTUMN PUMPKIN-CRANBERRY BREAD

In the fall, nut breads are one of my favorite things to serve as snacks, as appetizers, or with breakfast. This one is moist, easy, and delicious served warm. This bread also freezes easily.

Ingredients:

- 2 eggs
- ¾ c. honey
- ½ c. extra-virgin, pure coconut oil, plus more for pan
- ¼ c. ghee or softened butter
- 1 tsp. vanilla extract (or 1 vanilla bean, scraped)
- 1 T. orange peel, grated
- 1 c. pumpkin puree
- 1 c. whole-wheat flour
- 1 c. quinoa flour
- 3 tsp. baking powder
- 1 tsp. baking soda
- 1 tsp. cinnamon (ground)
- ¼ tsp. nutmeg (ground)
- ¼ tsp. ginger (ground)
- ¼ tsp. sea salt
- 1 c. cranberries (fresh), chopped
- ¾ c. walnuts, coarsely chopped

Directions:

1. Preheat oven to 350 degrees.
2. Grease a loaf pan with coconut oil and line with parchment paper.
3. Beat eggs until creamy in a medium bowl.
4. Add honey, coconut oil, butter, vanilla, orange peel, and pumpkin puree to egg mixture, and beat well.
5. In a large bowl, sift together flours, baking powder, baking soda, cinnamon, nutmeg, ginger, and salt.
6. Fold egg mixture into flour mixture.
7. Add cranberries and walnuts.
8. Pour batter into pan, and bake 50–60 minutes.
9. Cool about 15 minutes before taking out of the pan.

Note:

Check bread when it has been baking about 50 minutes. Insert a toothpick into the very middle of the bread. If it comes out clean, then bread is ready.

Variation:

Substitute raisins for cranberries.

GLUTEN-FREE FLOUR BLEND

This mixture will make a little over 4 cups of flour. Use it in recipes that call for gluten-free flour.

Ingredients:

1½ c. quinoa flour
1½ c. cornstarch or potato starch
1 c. tapioca flour
½ c. almond flour

Directions:

1. Mix all ingredients.

Raw recipe

LIVING CRACKERS

These are "raw" crackers that need to be made with a dehydrator. They are really yummy. I like to eat them when they are fresh out of the dehydrator. Surprisingly enough, I made these once and shared them with my brother, who is not a raw foodist or vegetarian, and he still talks about how great they are.

Ingredients:

2½ c. flax seeds
¼ c. chia seeds
½ c. red bell pepper, chopped
½ c. cilantro (fresh), chopped
1 c. sun-dried tomatoes
1½ c. tomatoes, chopped
1½ tsp. fresh jalapeno
3 cloves garlic, minced
pinch of mesquite spice
pinch of cayenne pepper
1 tsp. sea salt
2 T. extra-virgin olive oil or extra-virgin, pure coconut oil
1 tsp. honey (optional)

Directions:

1. Soak flax seeds in water overnight or at least 3 hours, and then drain off water.
2. Combine all ingredients (including honey, if using), except flax seeds, in a food processor and blend.
3. In a large bowl, combine flax seeds with mixture from food processor.
4. Coat dehydrator sheets with a tiny bit of coconut oil.
5. Spread cracker mixture onto solid dehydrator sheets in a thin layer.

6. Dehydrate at 90 to 116 degrees 4 hours or longer.
7. Gently remove crackers from solid dehydrator sheets and move to waffle-type dehydrating sheet (that let the air move through them).
8. Dehydrate another 4 hours, or until they are dry and a little crispy.

Variation:

Substitute pickled jalapeño for fresh.

PINEAPPLE-WALNUT MUFFINS

These delicious muffins are a variation from an old recipe from my Great-Aunt Alma. I used her pineapple upside-down cake recipe and changed it a bit. I use non-gluten flour for this and it works just great. These muffins are delicious served warm or room temperature.

Ingredients:

- 2 T. honey
- 1 c. walnuts, chopped
- 2 c. pineapple, in small chunks
- 1½ T. extra-virgin, pure coconut oil, melted
- 4 T. butter, melted
- 1 c. quinoa flour, sifted
- ¼ tsp. sea salt
- 2 tsp. baking powder
- 3 eggs, beaten well
- 4 T. raw sugar, xylitol, or date sugar (raw, organic)
- 5 T. pineapple juice

Directions:

1. Preheat oven to 350 degrees.
2. Put a little coconut oil in the bottom of each muffin cup or whatever pan that you are using. Cover the bottom with parchment paper (both sides coated with coconut oil).
3. Place honey, walnuts, pineapple, coconut oil, and butter in a small mixing bowl and combine well.
4. Put this mixture in equal amounts in the bottom of pan or muffin cups.
5. Sift together flour, sea salt, and baking powder.
6. Combine eggs, sugar, and pineapple juice.
7. Add egg mixture to flour mixture, and blend.
8. Pour pineapple-nut mixture in the muffin cups.

9. Bake about 30 minutes.

Variations:

1. Substitute wheat flour or oat flour for quinoa flour.
2. Substitute any type of granulated raw sugar.

SOUTHERN CORNBREAD

I grew up eating cornbread. I love it. This recipe is fairly quick and easy, and it pairs well with soup. If you use quinoa flour, it is gluten-free.

Ingredients:

2 T. extra-virgin, pure coconut oil
1 c. whole cornmeal
½ c. quinoa flour
1½ T. baking powder (non-aluminum)
½ tsp. baking soda
½ tsp. sea salt
2 eggs
1½ c. buttermilk
2 T. ghee, melted
2 T. honey

Directions:

1. Preheat oven to 450 degrees.
2. Place coconut oil in a 9-inch pan. Let oil melt in oven a couple of minutes. Remove from oven and set aside.
3. Sift together cornmeal, flour, baking powder, baking soda, and sea salt.
4. In a large bowl, beat eggs.
5. Add buttermilk, melted ghee, coconut oil from the pan (leaving a little bit in the pan), and honey to beaten eggs, and beat together.
6. Place a piece of parchment paper, cut to the size of the bottom of the pan, in the bottom of the pan. Coat with coconut oil and turn over, so both sides of parchment paper are lightly coated with coconut oil.
7. Add dry ingredients to wet ingredients and stir lightly.
8. Pour batter into prepared pan.
9. Bake 30–35 minutes. (The top should be golden brown and the sides should have pulled away from the sides of the pan.)

Note:

I always use parchment paper instead of aluminum foil. Aluminum is linked to many diseases, and it is best not to use it with food at all.

Leaving the parchment in the bottom of the baking pan will make it easier to remove when the bread finishes baking.

TEXAS BISCUITS

I grew up in Texas with a family of Southern cooks. Biscuits were a favorite bread served with many meals. Here is an easy recipe. Gluten-free flour works well in this recipe.

Biscuit are delicious reheated later, or buttered and broiled.

Ingredients:

1 T. yeast
2 T. warm water
3 T. honey
4½–5 c. sifted whole-grain flour (measured after sifting)
3 T. baking powder (aluminum-free)
1 tsp. baking soda
1 tsp. sea salt
1 c. extra-virgin, pure coconut oil
2 c. buttermilk

Directions:

1. Dissolve yeast in warm water and honey. Set aside.
2. Sift together flour, baking powder, baking soda, and sea salt.
3. Cut coconut oil into dry ingredients.
4. Combine yeast and buttermilk.
5. Add yeast-buttermilk mixture to dry ingredients.
6. Roll dough out onto floured board. Roll about 1/2-inch thick.
7. Use a biscuit cutter to cut out biscuits. Place each biscuit on a cookie sheet right next to each other. Cover with a clean cloth.
8. Let biscuits sit in a warm place about 45 minutes.
9. Bake in a preheated 400-degree oven 12–15 minutes. (They should be lightly golden brown on the top and bottom.)

Note:

Biscuits can be placed in a refrigerator or freezer on the cookie sheet, after they are baked. Wrap tightly with plastic or parchment paper and then foil, so they don't get freezer burn. Then they can be thawed completely and warmed up in a 350-degree oven 4–5 minutes.

WHOLE-GRAIN, GLUTEN-FREE BREAD

This is quick and easy bread, because it does not contain yeast.

Ingredients:

¼ c. extra-virgin, pure coconut oil (liquid, at room temperature)
2 eggs, beaten well
1 tsp. vanilla
1 c. milk
1 tsp. lemon peel, grated
2½ c. Gluten-Free Flour Blend (recipe on page 254)
1½ tsp. xanthan gum
1 tsp. vegetarian gelatin powder (or agar flakes)
2½ tsp. baking powder
1 tsp. sea salt
2/3 c. raw sugar or xylitol

Directions:

1. Preheat oven to 375 degrees.
2. Grease two loaf pans and line with parchment paper.
3. Beat coconut oil, eggs, vanilla, milk, and lemon peel until smooth.
4. Sift together Flour Blend, xanthan gum, gelatin powder, baking powder, sea salt, and sugar.
5. Add wet ingredients to dry ingredients. Combine quickly and gently.
6. Pour batter into baking pans quickly. Fill about halfway.
7. Bake about 35 minutes. (The top should be a light brown.)
8. Remove from oven and cool 15 minutes before removing from pans.

Variation:

Add ¼ c. each chopped nuts and grated apples.

Desserts

Sorbets

It is easy to make a healthy sorbet if you have a good blender. The only thing you need is really good fruit that you like. You blend it to a crème, and you can add a little coconut water, water, or a fruit juice to make it a bit thinner, or add another flavor to the creamy mixture. Vanilla beans can be scraped and added, or you can simply use vanilla extract or almond extract to add flavor.

A pound of fruit will yield two to three servings of sorbet. To add a nut flavor to a sorbet, soak the nuts overnight and then add them to the mixture. The nuts will cream better if they are soaked. Soaking will also make the nuts more digestible.

For someone who needs more nutritional impact or calories in his or her diet, add a teaspoon or two of raw, extra-virgin, pure coconut oil or coconut oil with the coconut meat in it to the mixture, a teaspoon or two of lecithin granules, a teaspoon of maca root powder, or a half-teaspoon of bee pollen. These four things would really boost the nutritional impact of the sorbet without really changing the flavor.

Here are a few recipes that you can use as guidelines for creating your own sorbet delights.

Raw recipe

CHERRY-ALMOND-VANILLA SORBET

Ingredients:

2 c. almonds, soaked overnight in enough water to cover them by ½ inch
1½ c. cherries
2 golden delicious apples, cored and peeled
1 vanilla bean (see note on page 262) or 2 T. vanilla extract
¼ c. apple juice, 2 T. raw honey or maple syrup, or ¼ tsp. liquid stevia
pinch of sea salt

Directions:

1. Blend all ingredients in food processor until smooth and creamy.
2. Place in a shallow pan and place in freezer until firm.

Note:

Split vanilla bean open and scrape out the inside to use. Discard shell.

Variations:

1. Substitute pistachios for almonds.
2. Substitute bananas for apples.

Raw recipe

CHERRY-CHOCOLATE SORBET

Ingredients:

2 c. cherries
2 T. honey
2 T. cacao nibs
¼–½ c. coconut water or milk of choice
pinch of sea salt

Directions:

1. Blend all ingredients in food processor until smooth and creamy.
2. Place in a shallow pan and place in freezer until firm.

Variation:

Add ½ c. raw cashews that have been soaked overnight (12 to 18 hours) in 1 c. water (coconut or regular) instead of coconut water or milk.

Raw recipe

PEACH SORBET

Ingredients:

1 lb. peaches, peeled, pitted, and sliced
1 c. ice
¼–½ c. fresh orange juice

Directions:

1. Blend all ingredients in food processor until smooth and creamy.
2. Add orange juice as needed to get a nice, smooth, creamy consistency.
3. Place in a shallow pan and place in freezer until firm.

Variation:

Substitute apricot nectar or another fruit juice for orange juice.

Raw recipe

ALMOND COOKIES

I frequently make these living-food cookies using almond meal I have leftover after making almond milk. I never wanted to waste the almond meal, and this is a wonderful way to use it. You can make these into small snack bars as well.

Store these cookies in the refrigerator.

Ingredients:

- 2 c. almonds, soaked in water 12 to 18 hours, or almond meal
- ½–1 tsp. sea salt
- ½ c. or more honey
- ¼ c. almond butter
- 2 T. protein powder
- ½ c. organic, raw, shredded coconut

Directions:

1. Grind almonds and sea salt into a fine meal.
2. Slowly add honey, almond butter, and protein powder to make sticky dough.
3. Roll dough into round long logs.
4. Roll logs in coconut.
5. Wrap logs in parchment or wax paper and then in foil.
6. Chill until firm.
7. Cut slices a little over one-quarter-inch thick.

Note:

I use Garden of Life brand protein powder.

Variation:

Gently press cookies in coconut after they are sliced, for a more coconut-y flavor.

Raw recipe

CASHEW CRÈME

Ingredients:

- ½ c. cashews, soaked overnight in water that just covers the top of the nuts
- ¼ c. water
- 2–5 drops liquid stevia

Directions:

1. Blend all ingredients in blender until creamy. Adjust the amount of water to make it thicker or thinner.

Note:

I like Sweet Leaf brand stevia that comes in flavors like English toffee and vanilla.

Variation:

Substitute nut milk for water.

Raw recipe

CHOCOLATE PIE FILLING OR PUDDING

Chocolate is the number-one anti-oxidant food in the world. It is the super-food of super-foods. It was widely used in food by the Mayan and Aztec cultures. When the Spanish arrived in North America, they learned of it and took it back to Europe with them. Cacao was used to treat fatigue, fever, and nervous disorders, and as a stimulant. The bean itself is extremely healthful; it is usually the added ingredients that can make the cacao unhealthy. The cacao bean is a dark purple-ish color and can be bitter in flavor. This is one of the reasons so much sugar is added to it in order to make sweet chocolate.

Serve this chilled with a dollop of flavored Cashew Crème (recipe on page 263) on top. Sometimes I serve this as a pudding, without the pie crust. Chocolate pudding is one of my favorite desserts. I made this for my mother and she loved it. She was so surprised when she found out the ingredients that she made it for her music club meeting luncheon as dessert.

Ingredients:

- 5 dates, pitted and soaked in water overnight
- 4 T. maple syrup (pure)
- ½ tsp. vanilla
- 2 avocados, pitted and peeled
- 1/3 c. cacao powder, raw and pure
- ¼ tsp. sea salt
- 1/3 c. milk
- 1 banana, sliced (optional)
- 1 Raw Pie Crust (recipe on page 267)

Directions:

1. Blend all ingredients except banana and Raw Pie Crust in food processor until creamy.
2. Add more milk as necessary. (You want a creamy, thick, and smooth consistency.)
3. Place sliced banana, if using, around the bottom of Raw Pie Crust.
4. Pour filling over banana slices.
5. Refrigerate at least 1 hour.

Note:

Almond or rice milk works well in this recipe.

Variation:

Serve as a pudding.

Raw recipe

FRUIT COOKIES

I used to make these in college. I've adjusted the recipe over the years; you can play with the ingredients. I didn't know what "raw food" was then, but I was doing raw food without knowing it. These cookies are not baked. Start these cookies the night before so that the fruit and nuts can be thoroughly softened by the time you want to make them. These cookies are easy to make if you have all of the ingredients and the time to start them the night before. They are also easy to chew and can really satisfy a sweet tooth. Keep cookies in the refrigerator for four to five days, or freeze them.

Ingredients:

- 5–6 figs (fresh or dried)
- 1 c. raisins
- 2 c. sunflower seeds
- 2 c. walnuts
- 1 c. purified water (from soaking ingredients overnight)
- 4 c. pineapple chunks (fresh)
- 1 c. mango chunks (fresh)
- 2 T. raw honey or maple syrup
- 1 T. chia seeds
- 1 T. sesame seeds
- 1 c. almond butter
- 1 tsp. extra-virgin, pure coconut oil
- ¼ tsp. sea salt
- ½ c. fruit juice
- 1 c. coconut (shredded)

Directions:

1. Soak figs and raisins in one bowl, and sunflower seeds and walnuts in a separate bowl overnight in purified water in the refrigerator.
2. Retain at least 1 cup water from figs and raisins to add to the recipe.
3. Discard all of the water used for soaking the nuts and seeds. Retain only one cup of the water used for soaking the figs and raisins.
4. Blend all ingredients except coconut in a food processor.
5. Using a teaspoon, scoop dough and roll into balls.
6. Roll balls in shredded coconut.
7. Place cookies on a dish and gently flatten.

Notes:

1. Sprouted nuts and seeds have a more vibrant nutritional value.
2. Good juice choices for this recipe are fresh papaya, apple, pear, and peach.
3. Using the soaking water in the recipe makes the cookie sweeter and less watery, as the water is sweeter.

Variations:

1. If you want a more traditional cookie and you have a dehydrator, place cookies on the flat sheets and dehydrate under 115 degrees for around 4 hours.
2. Substitute peanut butter for almond butter.
3. Substitute dates for raisins.
4. For extra nutrition, add a teaspoon of bee pollen, lecithin, kelp, and maca root powder, or even a little raw protein powder.

Raw recipe

OATMEAL PECAN COOKIES

I love oatmeal cookies. If you buy oatmeal that is not contaminated with gluten, these are gluten-free cookies! I add Garden of Life brand protein powder to add a little extra nutrition to them. I made these as a no-cook version of my old recipe, raw-food style!

Ingredients:

2 c. oats (raw)
1 tsp. raw protein powder
2/3 c. maple syrup
2 dates, soaked overnight in water
2 bananas
¾ c. pecans, chopped

Directions:

1. Combine oats, protein powder, maple syrup, dates, and bananas in food processor, and blend until you have a nice texture for cookie dough.
2. Add pecans and pulse gently. (Leave nuts in a chopped texture.)
3. Make teaspoon-sized balls of dough and drop onto a sheet for a dehydrator or a cookie sheet kind of dish.
4. Flatten each with a fork just a bit.
5. Dehydrate about 12 hours under 118 degrees, flip over, and dehydrate another 10 to 12 hours or overnight. If you don't have a dehydrator, simply place in refrigerator to firm up a little.

Note:

If you are not dehydrating these, leave them as cookie balls. They are easier to eat that way.

Variation:

Substitute walnuts for pecans.

Raw recipe

RAW PIE CRUST

Ingredients:

2 c. walnuts (raw)
1/8 tsp. sea salt (optional)
1½ c. dried apricots, chopped (non-sulfured)

Directions:

1. Combine walnuts and sea salt, if using, and grind in food processor.
2. Add apricots and continue to process until you have a dough-type consistency.
3. Press into a pie pan.
4. Cover pie shell and chill crust.
5. Fill pie with filling of choice and serve.

Notes:

1. If you wish to soak walnuts in order to help remove the phytic acid, soak them and then dehydrate them before using, or use the dehydrator after you have the pie crust in the pie pan.
2. If you have a dehydrator, dehydrate this pie shell 3 hours under 118 degrees, for a firmer crust, before you chill it. It is fine if you don't dehydrate it.
3. This crust can be frozen.

Variation:

You can use this pie crust recipe to make appetizers. Instead of putting the dough in a pie dish, roll it into little bite-sized balls for easy-to-eat snacks. Keep refrigerated for freshness.

"If slaughter houses had glass walls, every-one would be a vegetarian."

~ Paul McCartney

Part III
Natural Remedies

Growing up, I learned natural remedies from various people in my life. Many of these remedies have been passed down from generation to generation. Traditional natural remedies are a cherished and valued part of almost all cultures around the world. I have created a few of my own, and learned some from research and also from my doctors. What I like the most about these is that they are drug-free. This section contains some that I think are both easy and valuable.

Bloody Nose

The air gets very dry when we use heaters in our homes, particularly in the winter. A humidifier can really help. Adding a little eucalyptus or tea tree oil to the water in the humidifier adds a touch of natural antibacterial properties to the moist air. It also smells really good.

You can also use a cotton swab to coat the inside of the nostril with coconut oil or olive oil. This will moisten the dry skin lining the nostril and help it to not dry out and crack.

Body Products and Therapeutic Hygiene

Body products are usually tested on animals or have ingredients in them that are toxic. This section contains some products that I have found to be better and/or made at home. You have many foods in your kitchen that are really easy, less expensive, and healthy to use in making your own beauty and bath products for your daily bathing routine. Making them yourself also ensures that products have not been tested on animals.

The skin is the largest organ of the body and readily absorbs the products you put on it. Products go straight to the blood vessels, which is one reason the medical community now puts medicine on patches. The quality of ingredients is important. Buy organic if you have a choice.

Face Cleansers and Moisturizers

Honey is a natural moisturizer and has antibacterial properties. I use honey as my daily face cleanser. I love it because it makes my skin feel so smooth. Honey can also be used as a moisturizing mask. Put it on and leave for 10 or 15 minutes, and then remove it with a warm, wet washcloth. Your skin will feel moist and clean.

Extra-virgin, pure coconut oil is extremely good for almost any skin but really good for dry skin. I use it on my face and whole body.

Sesame seed oil pulls toxins from the skin. You can use it on your face or whole body. It has a little bit of a smell compared to coconut oil.

Face Masks

Avocado and cucumber mashed and blended together make a wonderfully refreshing, nutrient-dense mask. Cucumber slices can also be placed over the eyes to reduce swelling and redness.

Honey makes a very soothing and hydrating mask. Note: You can mix it with some oatmeal and eggs for a really nutrient-dense mask. Scrub it off with a warm, wet washcloth to exfoliate as well.

Yogurt is very calming and will help reduce redness of the skin. It makes a wonderful, cooling facial mask. Note: You can mix honey and/or eggs into yogurt, too. I like to experiment with ingredients. Strawberries and/or other fruits can be very nice to mash up and add. Experiment and find one that you love with the food you have on hand at the moment!

Eyes

Warm, wet tea bags are great for reducing swollen, puffy eyes. The tannins in the tea work on the swelling. I use English breakfast or chamomile tea for this. I put a tea bag in a cup of warm water and let it sit for a moment.

I put an old, dark towel under my head (so my good towels don't get stained), then I gently place a warm tea bag over each eye for about 15 minutes. You can do this again if you need to. It feels great and is so relaxing.

Exfoliating

Combine almonds (ground into a meal) mixed with an equal amount of oatmeal, a little purified water or cucumber juice (enough liquid to make a nice paste), and some honey. Spread the mixture evenly on the skin and let dry. When it is dry, take a dry washcloth and rub the face to remove the mixture. This will exfoliate the dry, dead skin cells and clean out the pores. Then take a warm, wet washcloth, wash it off, and rinse well. Note: I use the almond meal I have leftover from making my almond milk for this!

Hair

Olive oil, coconut oil, or mayonnaise can be used to moisturize and condition hair. Put it on the hair and place a plastic cap on it overnight (or even just for an hour or so), and then wash in the morning.

Letting your hair naturally dry as often as you can really helps your hair and scalp. Using a hair dryer is also very drying and can cause brittle hair ends.

Body Scrubs, Moisturizers, Baths, and Foot Baths

Sea salt, a few drops of an essential oil of your choosing, like eucalyptus or peppermint, and a little olive oil make a wonderful body scrub to remove dead skin and improve circulation. You can use sugar instead of sea salt.

For a nice bath or foot soak, put some mineral salts or sea salts in the bath with a little organic apple cider vinegar (to help adjust the pH balance of your body), and fill the tub with warm water. Right before you get in, add a few drops of eucalyptus oil and/or peppermint oil (to invigorate) or oil like lavender (to relax) to the bath or foot bath. Put the oil in at the last minute or it will dissipate, and you won't get to really enjoy the aromatic effect.

Coconut oil is extremely good for most skin types, especially dry skin. I use it on my whole body, including my face. You can add a few drops of your favorite essential oil to add a scent. (Note: I don't use the scented oil on my face, only on my body.) I also like to put coconut oil mixed with peppermint or lavender oil on my feet and then put some socks on for the night. These oils are really refreshing. The socks help soften and nourish the dry skin on the feet.

Castor oil pulls toxins from the body. It is thick and gooey, but I have gotten used to it and use it fairly regularly on my face and body after showering. After I put it on my skin, I just put on my nice, thick robe and socks for a little while before I get dressed.

I have been using oils for my skin for many years. I had a facialist put purifying oils on me a few times and I was hooked. I found that my skin felt so much better when I used natural oils instead of traditional lotions. Olive oil, pure coconut oil, jojoba oil, almond oil, and apricot oil all make wonderful body moisturizers/oils. Olive oil has a little fragrance. My daughter puts olive oil all over her body in the shower just before getting out, and then quickly does her last rinse. She loves the way it makes her skin feel, and she doesn't have oil on her skin after she has dried off, even though her skin feels nourished, hydrated, and soft. Be careful not to slip in the shower if you do this, as olive oil can make the shower floor slippery.

Dry Skin Brushing

Skin brushing can do wonders for the whole body, mind, and spirit. I have done this for over 20 years and raised my children doing it. Buy a natural bristle brush with a long handle, so you can reach body parts like the middle of your back. Wetting skin will not have the same effect. Try this for a week and see if you can get used to doing it.

Wonderful benefits from skin brushing include:

- Removing dead skin and cleaning out the pores of fresh skin.
- Tightening skin.
- Helping with digestion. (Since skin brushing stimulates the body muscles and the circulation system, it can also stimulate the body in continuing to move anything in the intestinal tract through the intestines.)
- Removing cellulite.
- Stimulating circulation.
- Increasing cell renewal.
- Strengthening the immune system.
- Stimulating and cleaning the lymphatic system and glands all over the body.

Try skin brushing every day before showering or bathing. Start with the feet. All of the body organs and nerve endings are connected to the feet, so when you treat the feet, you are also treating the whole body. You can work from the feet up the legs to the torso, and lastly the arms and hands.

When brushing, always work upward in counter-clockwise circles toward the heart. It is all right to do this lightly where you are more sensitive. After you take a warm shower or bath, rinse with cool water to seal up the skin and stimulate blood circulation. This will actually stimulate the surface warmth of the skin.

Wash the skin brush every week in water and let it dry before using again.

If you just can't do dry skin brushing, then try using a tough brush on your skin in the shower to really clean out the toxins and dirt from the pores. It will also help with circulation.

Hand Sanitizer/Hand Soap

Since antibiotic hand sanitizers have been on the market, many doctors believe they may be contributing to the development of super strains of viruses and bacteria. Also, they absorb right through our skin into our blood stream, so using an antibacterial soap or hand sanitizer is basically like taking an antibiotic. The antibiotic kills all bacteria, including the good bacteria in our body that keep the bad bacteria in check. These good bacteria are a main part of our immune system. Before antibiotics were invented, natural oils and foods were used to help protect the body from pathogens.

In a *New York Times* article about Dr. Lawrence D. Rosen, a New Jersey pediatrician who makes and sells natural health advice and remedies, Rosen recommended his recipe for a homemade hand sanitizer called thieves oil.[156] His mixture of oils came from a legend about a group of 15th-century European perfumers who started robbing bodies during the Bubonic Plague. They stole anything of value off of dead bodies. They made a mixture of essential oils that had antibacterial and antiviral properties, and covered their bodies with the mixture. They also used this oil on their bodies to protect themselves from the germs—hence the name "thieves oil." Dr. Rosen's recipe includes equal amounts of cinnamon bark, lemon, eucalyptus, clove, and rosemary therapeutic-grade essential oils. Mix the oils with coconut oil or jojoba oil as a carrier, and use it on hands as a sanitizer. For soap, you can mix it with a pure castile soap.

I use a mouthwash with this blend of oils in it as well. Essential oils are very potent. You may find it wise to do a skin test first, to make sure you don't have any adverse reactions to the oils of choice. In my opinion, these natural antibacterial oil combinations are a great, natural alternative to the "antibiotic" versions.

Hangover Cures

Cure #1:

Combine 1 tsp. honey, 1/2 c. orange juice, and ¼ c. kefir or yogurt, and consume.

Cure #2:

Soak dates in water for a few hours or more. Drink the water and eat the dates.

Cure #3:

Eat a banana.

Honey and Cinnamon

The combination of honey and cinnamon has been used for centuries for many ailments and problems. They both have powerful antibacterial properties. Canadian magazine *Weekly World News* listed the following diseases and conditions that can be cured by honey and cinnamon, according to research conducted by Western scientists: heart disease, insect bites, arthritis, hair loss, bladder infections, cholesterol, colds, infertility, upset stomach, gas, immune system issues, indigestion, longevity, pimples, skin infections, cancer, fatigue, bad breath, and hearing loss.[157]

Ceylon cinnamon is the best cinnamon to use. Cassia, Saigon, and Chinese cinnamon contain 5% coumarin, which is problematic for the liver. Ceylon cinnamon has only .0004% coumarin.

HONEY-CINNAMON DRINK

Ingredients:

1 T. honey

¼ c. lukewarm water

1 tsp. cinnamon

Directions:

Mix together all ingredients.

Note:

Drink on an empty stomach or before a meal.

SLEEP AID

Ingredients:

1 tsp. honey

1 c. warm milk or chamomile tea

Directions:

1. Mix ingredients together.

Kombucha Tea

Kombucha tea is gaining popularity throughout the world. Kombucha is a colony of bacteria and yeast. Kombucha tea is made by adding the colony to sugar and black or green tea, and allowing the mixture to ferment. The resulting liquid contains vinegar, B vitamins, and a number of other chemical compounds. Kombucha tea is commonly prepared by taking a starter sample from an existing culture and growing a new colony in a fresh jar. "Health benefits attributed to Kombucha tea include stimulating the immune system, preventing cancer, and improving digestion and liver function."[158]

Kombucha has been used in China for over 2,000 years. In ancient Chinese it is called the immortal health elixir. Kombucha is rich with B vitamins, anti-oxidants, glucaric acids, and glucosamines. German and Russian scientists began researching kombucha around the early 1900s.

Kombucha tea is a probiotic beverage that has been known to improve digestion and fight candida (harmful yeast) overgrowth and depression, as well as promote general health and well-being. You can buy kits to make your own or purchase it already made.

Nails and Cuticles

When you get out of the warm bath or shower and cuticles are soft and pliable, take your towel and gently push back each cuticle all the way around. This will keep cuticles back and healthy, and you won't need to cut or trim them as much. You can also use a wooden cuticle stick to do this. Rub some oil into cuticles to keep them soft and from drying out. (I use any of the oils that I use after showering, like coconut, almond, olive, apricot, and castor oil.) Do this after a bath or shower; it can help seal in the moisture.

Sore Throat and/or Stuffy Nose

My family went to Dr. Ludwig Michaels, an ear, nose, and throat doctor, for many years. He used a bulb syringe filled with a mixture of sea salt and warm water, inserted it into one nostril, and gently pressed the warm salt water into the nostril. The water would come out the other nostril, along with any congestion. He repeated that process on each side a couple of times. We held our head over a bowl to catch the water that came out. It always cleared up our congestion and was refreshing. Neti pots work in the same way, but I don't think they are as easy to use as a bulb syringe. You can buy rubber bulb syringes and neti pots at many pharmacies.

Sore Throat Remedies

#1

Mix 1 tsp. honey and 2 tsp. freshly squeezed lemon juice. Drink on an empty stomach, and then drink a glass of water 15–20 minutes later.

#2

Gargle with warm sea salt and water.

#3

Mash 1 garlic clove, let sit about 10 minutes, and then mix with some butter. Spread on a piece of bread or cracker and eat.

Sunscreen

We want to protect ourselves and our children from the sun during the summer, but what else is there to know about the sun, and what sunscreen should you use? Recent studies reveal that many sunscreens can cause Vitamin D3 deficiency, increase the risk of skin cancer, and take away the sun's benefits, such as access to Vitamin D.[159]

It is estimated that about 87% of the population is Vitamin D–deficient in the winter months, and that seven out of 10 children and 70% of breastfed babies are deficient in Vitamin D3, which affects their growth and development.[160] The sun promotes health and vitality. Because of these alarming numbers, many doctors recommend significant everyday supplements of Vitamin D and more specifically Vitamin D3. Vitamin D is actually a hormone, known as calcitriol in its active form. A deficiency of calcitriol may be responsible for over 17 cancers, autoimmune disease, multiple sclerosis, osteoarthritis, hypertension/high blood pressure, diabetes, depression, and genetic disorders, and may increase the risk of cardiovascular disease.[161] Rickets (bone softening) is a disease caused by Vitamin D deficiency. Sounds a lot like osteoporosis, doesn't it? If you have a bone problem, have your Vitamin D checked. That may be a big part of the problem.

The American Medical Association recommends we get at least 15 minutes of direct mid-day sun, without applying sunscreen, several times a week, yet the American Academy of Dermatology says "there is no scientifically validated, safe threshold level of UV exposure from the sun that allows for maximal vitamin D3 synthesis, without increasing skin cancer risk."[162] It is up to you to decide, but regardless, be sure not to stay out in the sun and burn from prolonged exposure. Humans have been getting their Vitamin D from the sun for centuries, and foods with Vitamin D are few and insufficient.

Most experts agree with the American Medical Association's recommendations for sun exposure. The amount of skin exposed to sunshine correlates directly with how much Vitamin D will be produced. The more skin exposed, the more Vitamin D will be created. Also, people with darker skin actually need more sunlight than lighter-skinned people. We also need sunlight through our eyes without sunglasses each day.

For about 25 years, we have used sunscreens that block out UVB rays, but not UVA rays. UVB rays were thought to be the cause of skin cancer, but studies now reveal that sunscreens were blocking UVB cancer-protecting rays and allowing in UVA rays that can cause cancer. There is no Vitamin D toxicity from sunshine, because UVA rays break down excess Vitamin D. We can store Vitamin D in fat cells and use it in the winter months if we get enough in the summer.

UVB rays are at their peak in the summer and are not available for most of the winter north of Atlanta, Georgia. When UVB rays stay on the skin surface they help the body make Vitamin D3, which is why they were incorrectly blamed for causing skin cancer. The SPF rating only measured the UVB blocking power. Sunscreens reportedly reduce Vitamin D3 levels in the blood by up to 99 percent.

What do you do about sunscreen if you need to be outside for long periods of time? Pick a safe sunscreen. Some sunscreens have carcinogenic ingredients and hormone disrupters that should be avoided: Oxtinoxate, Octisalate, Oxybenzone, Homosalate, Avobenzone, and Retinyl Palmitate (a form of Vitamin A). Be sure to check any sunscreens for these ingredients; they absorb easily through the skin and are toxic when combined with sun exposure. Zinc oxide and titanium dioxide are safe, active sunscreen ingredients to look for. They are not absorbed through the skin but reflect the sun's UVA and UVB rays.

The Environmental Workers Group (EWG) tested over 1,500 sunscreens for safety and effectiveness. The sunscreens listed below contain either zinc oxide or titanium dioxide in some form. The ones with a star by them are recommended as the safest.[163]

Thinkbaby and Thinksport **
UV Natural *
Soleo Organics *
Badger *
Loving Naturals *
Purple Prairie Botanicals *
Beyond Coastal
California Baby
Desert Essence
Episenical
Jason Natural Cosmetics
Estion
Caribbean Solutions
All Terrain
Kababa Skin Care
L'uvalla Certified Organic
Little Forest
Miessence
Trukid
Vanicream

UV Natural is a good sunscreen, and one of the safest. It contains 24.8% zinc oxide and green tea extract, grape seed, and macadamia nut oil.

Drinking carrot juice or eating carrots also gives the body some natural sun protection (from the beta carotene).

Tea Tree Oil for Poison Ivy, Bug Bites, Chicken Pox, Etc.

Tea tree oil has been a staple of my medicine cabinet ever since I started using it. The New Zealand variety smells better than the Australian type, in my opinion, but both work really well.

When my son was 4, he got chicken pox. He is a redhead and has very sensitive skin. I put tea tree oil on each spot all over his body. I thought it would help him to not itch or scratch. In the morning, his chicken pox were gone with no scars, no itching, and no complications. It was amazing. His doctor was completely amazed, as was his preschool teacher. I have used it on just about everything ever since.

One time my contractor had terrible poison ivy. He had used cortisone, medicines from the doctor, and everything he could think of for over four months. He was absolutely miserable. I gave him my tea tree oil to try. The next day, he came back absolutely amazed at how well it had worked on healing the poison ivy. His poison ivy was gone in a matter of days.

I use the oil any place that has a fluid in it. It also has antibacterial properties. You are not supposed to use it on an open wound.

Teeth, Gums, and Mouth

The mouth is highly absorbable. If you read the box of some name-brand toothpastes or mouthwashes, you may see a warning that if they are swallowed you should call poison control immediately. The warnings are usually only on the toothpaste box and not on the toothpaste tube itself. In my opinion, we shouldn't be putting any kind of poison in our mouths at all. I buy brands that are free of poison and not harmful to my body. I use an essential oil toothpaste and mouthwash.

Do not share your toothpaste. It can spread germs with others' toothbrushes brushing up on the end of the toothpaste opening.

Get a new toothbrush after any illness, or at least every two months. This will prevent the toothbrush from becoming too built up with germs.

Use a tongue scraper to keep the tongue clean and fresh. Also, floss at least once daily to keep gums healthy and to remove bacteria from between teeth.

Wheatgrass

The amazing health benefits of using wheatgrass for healing were brought to the public's attention by Ann Wigmore in *The Wheatgrass Book: How to Grow and Use Wheatgrass to Maximize Your Health and Vitality.* When I started learning about cleansing, some 25 years ago, I started learning about the amazing positive effects grasses have on our body. I learned about barley grass as well as wheatgrass. The chlorophyll-rich grasses have enormous amounts of anti-oxidants and are highly alkalizing. There are so many benefits for consuming juice freshly extracted from grasses. Here are some of the benefits, according to Ann Wigmore.[164]

Wheatgrass juice can:

- When externally applied to the skin, help eliminate itching almost immediately.
- Soothe sunburned skin and act as a disinfectant.
- When rubbed into the scalp before a shampoo, help mend damaged hair and alleviate itchy, scaly scalp conditions.
- Soothe and heal cuts, burns, scrapes, rashes, poison ivy, athlete's foot, insect bites, boils, sores, open ulcers, tumors, and so on. (Use as a poultice and replace every two to four hours.)
- Return gray hair to its natural color.
- Greatly increase energy levels when consumed daily.
- When the juice is consumed, act as a beauty treatment that slows down the aging process. Wheatgrass will cleanse your blood and help rejuvenate aging cells, slowing the aging process way down and making you feel more alive right away. It will help tighten loose and sagging skin.
- Lessen the effects of radiation. One enzyme found in wheatgrass, SOD, lessens the effects of radiation and acts as an anti-inflammatory compound that may prevent cellular damage following heart attacks or exposure to irritants.
- Restore fertility and promote youthfulness.
- Work as a sleep aid. Place a tray of living wheatgrass near the head of your bed. It will enhance the oxygen in the air and generate healthful negative ions to help you sleep more soundly.
- When gargled, sweeten the breath, and firm and tighten gums.

Many health clinics in the United States today (like the Ann Wigmore Foundation and Retreat Center, Hippocrates Institute, Tree of Life, and Optimum Clinic, just to name a few) use wheatgrass as a mainstay basic of their healing programs. The grass is high in anti-oxidants, oxygenates the blood, and is nutrient-dense. It is such an easy and simple healing modality.

"If man wants freedom, why he keeps birds and animals in cages? Truly man is the king of beasts, for his brutality exceeds them. We live by the death of others. We are buried places! I have since an early age, abjured the use of meat."

~ Leonardo da Vinci

A Closing Note

Writing this book has been such a joy for me. I have learned so much over the years and now find so much happiness in being able to share all of this information with you. May you find health and happiness with the vegetarian lifestyle! Bless you.

And remember: The main ingredient is always love!

~ Nancy

"There is no reason why animals should be slaughtered to serve as human diet, when there are so many substitutes man can live without meat."

~ The Dalai Lama

Resources

ACUPUNCTURE

Dr. Alan Chen
4100 W. 15th Street
Plano, TX 75075
(972) 599–0852

Dr. Chen is a medical doctor and orthopedist in China. He is a licensed acupuncturist and herbologist, and a licensed doctor of chiropractic medicine in the United States.

ALTERNATIVE HEALING INSTITUTES

The Hippocrates Institute
secure.hippocratesinst.org/

Optimum Health Institute
www.optimumhealth.org/locations/ohi-austin.htm

Tree of Life Rejuvenation Center
treeofliferejuvenationcenter.wordpress.com/tree-of-life-rejuvenation-center/

BLENDERS AND JUICERS

Breville Juicer
www.compare99.com/p/Breville-Juicers?p2=Juicers&gclid=CL2Zl9yalasCFVsS2godTQF5mw

This juicer is easy to use and pretty easy to clean as well. It is also comparatively low-priced. The Breville Juice Fountain boasts several features that other popular juice extractor brands simply don't have. This site has good prices for the Breville Juicer.

Vitamix
secure.vitamix.com/?COUPON=06-006525&store=1

Blendtec
www.blendtec.com/

This blender is easy to clean, powerful, and great for liquefying any food.

Lexen Juicers
www.lexenproducts.com

Discount Juicers
www.discountjuicers.com

Discount Juicers has a large selection of juicers for wheatgrass and various other fruits and vegetables, which often need different juicers for juicing. Some are manual and some are electric. The site has some information about the different juicers, and rates them.

BOOKS

ABC of Asthma, Allergies and Lupus: Eradicate Asthma—Now! by Dr. Fereydoon Batmanghelidj

Alive and Cooking by Maryann DeLeo and Nancy Addison

Alkalize or Die by Dr. Theodore A. Baroody

Anatomy of the Spirit by Caroline Myss, PhD

The Anti-Inflammation Zone by Dr. Barry Sears

Becoming Vegan: The Complete Guide to Adopting a Plant-Based Diet by Brenda Davis, RD, and Vesanto Melina, MS, RD

Blink by Malcolm Gladwell

The Cancer Solution by Robert Willner, MD, PhD

Candida Albicans: Could Yeast Be Your Problem? by Leon Chaitow, ND, DO

The Candle Café Cookbook by Joy Peirson and Bart Potenza, with Barbara Scott-Goodman

The China Study by T. Colin Campbell, PhD

Coconut Cures by Bruce Fife, ND

Complete Candida Yeast Guidebook: Everything You Need to Know About Prevention, Treatment & Diet, Revised 2nd Edition by Jeanne Marie Martin and Zoltan P. Rona, MD

Daylight Robbery: The Importance of Sunlight to Health by Dr. Damien Downing

Diet for a New America by John Robbins

Eat, Drink and Be Healthy by Walter C. Willett, MD

Enzyme Nutrition: The Food Enzyme Concept by Dr. Edward Howell

Enzymes for Health and Longevity by Dr. Edward Howell

Excitotoxins: The Taste That Kills by Dr. Russell L. Blaylock

Fast Food Nation by Eric Schlosser

Food and Healing by Annemarie Colbin

Food for Life by Neal Barnard, MD

The Food Revolution by John Robbins

Foods That Fight Pain by Neal Barnard, MD

Genetic Roulette by Jeffrey Smith

Heal Your Body by Louise L. Hay

Healing with Whole Foods by Paul Pritchard

Health and Nutrition Secrets That Can Save Your Life by Dr. Russell L. Blaylock

The Hippocrates Diet and Health Program by Dr. Ann Wigmore

How to Deal With Back Pain and Rheumatoid Joint Pain by Dr. Fereydoon Batmanghelidj

Light, Radiation and You: How to Stay Healthy by John Ott

Listen from the Inside Out: An Everyday Guide to the Secrets of Sound Healing by Sharon Carne

Living on Live Food by Alissa Cohen

The McDougall Program for a Healthy Heart: A Live-Saving Approach to Preventing and Treating Heart Disease by John A. McDougall, MD; recipes by Mary McDougall

The Message from Water by Masaru Emoto

The Natural Hygiene Handbook by the American Natural Hygiene Society

Natural Strategies for the Cancer Patient by Dr. Russell Blaylock

Obesity Cancer & Depression: Their Common Cause & Natural Cure by Dr. Fereydoon Batmanghelidj

Prescription for Nutritional Healing: A Practical A–Z Reference to Drug-Free Remedies Using Vitamins, Minerals, Herbs & Food Supplements, 3rd Edition by Phyllis A. Balch, CNC

Program for Reversing Heart Disease: The Only System Scientifically Proven to Reverse Heart Disease Without Drugs or Surgery by Dr. Dean Ornish

Raw: The Uncook Book by Juliano

The Raw Food Detox Diet by Natalia Rose

Raw Food for Everyone: Essential Techniques and 300 Simple-to-Sophisticated Recipes by Alissa Cohen with Leah J. Dubois

The Secret Life of Water by Masaru Emoto

Skinny Bitch and Skinny Bastard by Rory Freedman and Kim Barnouin

Staying Healthy with Nutrition: The Complete Guide to Diet and Nutritional Medicine by Elson M. Haas, MD

The Sunfood Diet Success System by David Wolfe

There Is a Cure for Diabetes by Gabriel Cousens, MD

Water: For Health, for Healing, for Life: You're Not Sick, You're Thirsty! by Dr. Fereydoon Batmanghelidj

Water Crystal Healing by Masaru Emoto

Water Cures: Drugs Kill: How Water Cured Incurable Diseases by Dr. Fereydoon Batmanghelidj

You Can Heal Your Life by Louise L. Hay

You'll See it When You Believe It by Dr. Wayne Dyer

Your Body's Many Cries for Water by Dr. Fereydoon Batmanghelidj

CANCER RESOURCES

Stanislaw R. Burzynski, MD, PhD

www.burzynskiclinic.com

Dr. Burzynski is an internationally recognized physician and biochemical researcher who has a clinic to diagnose, prevent, and treat cancer patients.

Dr. Johanna Budwig

www.budwigcenter.com/

Dr. Budwig was one of Germany's top biochemists as well one of the best cancer researchers throughout all of Europe.

CHIROPRACTOR

Dr. Michael W. Hall, DC, CCST, DABCN, FIACN

hallchiropracticwellnesscenter.chiromatrixbase.com/custom_content/c_23295_contact_us.html?hallchiropracticwellnesscenter_com=5309h9a2rpi3voos20l4phtdd6

(972) 304–3900

Dr. Hall is a chiropractic neurologist. Along with his wife, Cara, who is also a chiropractor trained in clinical neurology and therapeutic massage, they run the Hall Chiropractic and Family Wellness Center in Dallas and in Coppell, Texas.

CLEANSING

Detox & Cleanse

www.detox.net.au/articles/detoxification.html

This is a good site for finding various cleansing products, including bentonite clay.

Yerba Prima

www.yerba.com/

DIGESTIVE ENZYMES

Garden of Life enzymes

www.organichealthylifestyle.com (order from my website)

Dr. Mercola Digestive Enzymes

products.mercola.com/digestive-enzymes/

ESSENTIAL OILS

Spiritual Creations TM

www.spiritualcreationsoils.com

c/o Miracles of Joy

701 S. Old Orchard Lane, Suite C

Lewisville, TX 75067

(972) 221–8080

E-mail: Larry@spiritualcreationsoils.com

Larry with Spiritual Creations makes wonderful essential oils blends to wear as perfume. I have been wearing his blends for many years. Many people comment on the wonderful fragrance.

Young Living Oils

www.organic healthylifestyle.com (order from my website)

I use a variety of the oils from this company.

Their "Thieves" mouthwash and cleaning products are really great.

I have been using their mouthwash for over 15 years.

GROCERY STORES

Whole Foods Market

www.wholefoodsmarket.com

This is my favorite store for grocery shopping. They were the first nationally certified organic grocer in the United States. I understand that this store tries very hard to keep quality at the most optimum level, and that they stand by their products. Because they stand by their products, they have a wonderful return policy. Whole Foods Market also has their 365 brand products, which are usually less expensive than other products. I asked an employee one day about the 365 products that are not labeled organic. She researched it and told me that Whole Foods Market makes every attempt to use only non–genetically modified foods in all of their products, if at all possible.

They have locations all over the United States, in Canada, and in the United Kingdom. They usually have a large takeout area, as well as a bakery, for anyone needing to pick up freshly made food to go.

Sprouts

sprouts.com/content.php?frameSrc=http://sprouts.com/press/

This store sells organic produce and products. It is based in Arizona and has stores in California, Texas, Colorado, and Arizona.

Sunflower Market

www.sunflowermarkets.com/Mission.aspx

Sunflower Market sells some organic produce and products, often at a great price. They have about 40 stores in Texas, California, Oklahoma, New Mexico, Arizona, Utah, Nevada, and Colorado.

Natural Grocers

www.naturalgrocers.com/store-info/store-directory/texas

This store sells organic produce and products, often at great prices.

They have locations in Idaho, Kansas, Missouri, Nebraska, New Mexico, Oklahoma, Texas, Utah, and Wyoming.

New Frontiers

newfrontiersmarket.com/

This store is a supporter of non–genetically modified foods. I have found some really nice organic produce and products at this market. They have locations in Arizona and California.

Trader Joes

www.traderjoes.com/about/our-story.asp

They carry some organic produce and products at this market. Their private label is from non–genetically modified sources.

HAIRCUT

A great haircut can make a person feel fantastic.

Roy Teeluck

royteeluck.com/
5 East 57th St.
New York, NY 10022
(212) 888–2221

200 S. Biscayne Blvd., Suite 700 A
Miami, Fl 33131
(305) 372–1278

HEALTH COUNSELOR SCHOOL

The Institute of Integrative Nutrition

www.integrativenutrition.com/

I went to this school and loved it! It was one of the best experiences I have had. If you choose to enroll, tell them you heard about the school from me!

HEALTHFUL COOKING SCHOOLS

The Natural Gourmet Institute

naturalgourmetinstitute.com/

48 W. 21st St., 2nd Floor
New York, NY 10010
(212) 645–5170

The Natural Gourmet Institute offers classes year-round to the public. There are a variety of classes on health, supportive culinary arts, and theory.

They also have a wonderful chef training program.

Alissa Cohen

www.alissacohen.com/

Alissa teaches and certifies people in raw and living foods.

I was certified as a raw food chef by Alissa.

KITCHEN SUPPLIES

Williams- Sonoma

www.williams-sonoma.com/

This store has a good selection of high-quality kitchen tools and equipment.

Sur la Table

www.surlatable.com

This store has a good selection of high-quality kitchen tools and equipment.

Real Goods

www.realgoods.com/product/09-9115.do

Recycled and PBA-free containers. Good source for plastic bowls.

MAIL-ORDER FOODS

Natalia Rose/Detox the World

www.detoxtheworld.com/

Natalia sells food for delivery just about anywhere. She is located in New York City. She has other resources for juicing, detoxing, colonics, etc. She has great books and recipes. Her site is an awesome resource.

Veggie Brothers

www.veggiebrothers.com
(877) 834–2655

This is a 100% vegan/vegetarian online store. Veggie Brothers uses the best and freshest natural and organic ingredients available. None of their ingredients have been genetically modified.

Raw Guru

www.rawguru.com/store/raw-food/nama-shoyu-raw-organic-

Raw food to order online.

Local Harvest

www.localharvest.org/

Organic Authority

www.organicauthority.com/

This website can help you locate locally grown, organic foods.

MAIL-ORDER FOODS AND FOODS FOUND IN GROCERY STORES

Pacific Foods

www.pacificfoods.com

Almond milk. (I like unsweetened vanilla.) This company has some great soups that are low in sugar, which is a better option for anyone with diabetes. But be sure to read ingredient lists, because some soups are higher in sugar. Nonetheless, they have some really good choices for store-bought foods.

Fig Food Company

figfood.com/

This company has a variety of products. They have BPA-free packaging. One of their products is soup. The Tuscan white bean soup only has 1 gram of sugar in it.

Amy's

www.amys.com

This company has a variety of frozen meals and foods. Amy's cheese pizza is delicous. I served it when my children had slumber parties and other occasions when I needed fast, easy, and healthy food for more "mainstream" people. Amy's also has some burgers and other meat alternatives. Although they are not totally organic and they have soy in them, they are good to have if you are simply craving some transition food from being a carnivore. I like the Texas Burger best. This is the type of burger that I take when I am invited to a cookout and need to take my own food.

Seeds of Change

www.seedsofchange.com

This company makes wonderful, high-quality, organic food products.

Tru Roots

www.truroots.com/

This company has a variety of products including sprouted whole grains in bulk.

Shiloh Farms

www.shilohfarms.com

This is a good brand for bulk, organic whole grains.

Bob's Red Mill

www.bobsredmill.com

Bob's Red Mill is carried at most healthy grocery stores, and they sell a variety of healthy grains and flours.

Arrowhead Mills

www.arrowheadmills.com/

This company has a variety of products including organic oat bran.

Alvarado Street Bakery

www.alvaradostreetbakery.com/index.html

This company makes delicious organic, whole-grain breads. Outside of California, their breads can be found in the freezer section of the market. Alvarado Street Bakery is located just north of San Francisco in Sonoma County. Their products are sold in the United States, Canada, and Japan.

Food for Life

www.foodforlife.com

Their almond Ezekiel 4.9 Sprouted Whole Grain Cereal is one of my favorites.

They also have a variety of breads that are delicious.

Tinkyana Rice Pasta

www.nextag.com/tinkyada-rice-pasta/compare-html?nxtg=7c750a24051b-CF63729B7EA53C31

This brand is very good for a gluten-free pasta. It's made from certified organic whole-grain rice and does not become mushy when cooked, if you don't cook it too long.

Bionaturae

www.bionaturae.com

This is a resource for whole-grain, certified organic pasta.

DeBoles Organic and All-Natural Pastas

www.deboles.com/

My daughter and I love their spelt pasta.

Annie's Organic

www.Annies.com

My kids love their shells with real aged cheddar. Though some of their products are made with whole-grain ingredients, note that others are not.

Doctor Kracker

www.drkracker.com

These are organic, whole-grain crackers in a variety of flavors.

Mary's Gone Crackers

www.marysgonecrackers.com

These crackers are organic, kosher, non-GMO, whole-grain, vegan, and wheat-free; contain no hydrogenated oils; and are manufactured in a gluten-free, dairy-free, nut-free facility.

Wholly Wholesome

www.whollywholesome.com

They make organic whole-wheat or spelt pie crust shells.

Sun Warrior

www.sunwarrior.com/products/sunwarrior-ormusgreens

They make power-packed, raw, and organic green concentrated food powder, as well as protein powders.

Sensational Sea Salt Seasoning

www.sensationalseasaltseasoning.com

Sensational Sea Salt Seasoning is patent pending and created by Nancy Addison. This proprietary seasoning blend of mineral and nutrient dense, whole, raw, organic food made up of the finest sea salts, sea kelps, and omega 3 and Vitamin E rich seeds to boost the absorption of the iodine from the ingredients, which is the main nutrient that supports the thyroid gland. Use in place of your normal salt.

Yerba Prima

www.yerbaprima.com

These kalenite cleansing herbs and psyllium husks are a great source of fiber and good for digestive health.

Organic Ville Foods

organicvillefoods.com/products/condiments/stone-ground-organic-mustard/

Organic stone-ground mustard.

Hain Safflower Mayonnaise

www.hainpurefoods.com/index.php

Sweet Leaf

www.sweetleaf.com/

Makers of SweetLeaf Sweetener®

1203 W. San Pedro St.

Gilbert, AZ 85233

(480) 921–1373

(800) 899–9908

Source for stevia sugar alternative.

Now

www.nowfoods.com

Brand of xylitol.

Maine Coast Sea Vegetables

www.seaveg.com

Certified organic sea kelp is a great source of iodine in a whole-food form and other nutrients! Dulse Flakes are easily ready to sprinkle into dishes or use in recipes.

Gold Mine Natural Food Co.

www.goldminenaturalfood.com

Nama Shoyu raw, organic soy sauce is raw, organic, non–genetically modified, and aged four years.

Braggs Soy Sauce

www.bragg.com

Braggs is a company that makes wonderful organic soy sauce and apple cider vinegar, as well as other products.

Teeccino Caffé, Inc.
teeccino.com/category/11/Herbal-Coffees.html
P.O. Box 40829
Santa Barbara, CA 93140
(800) 498–3434
(805) 966–0999 (outside the US and Canada)
Coffee alternatives.

Garden of Life: Vitamins, Protein Powders, Green Food Powders, etc.
www.organichealthylifestyle.com or www.gardenoflife.com
Garden of Life has vitamins, snack bars, green foods,, meal substitutes and protein powders that are raw, certified organic, gluten-free, and vegan.

Pomona's Universal Pectin
www.pomonapectin.com
This is what I use to make Jell-O type foods. Recipes can be found on the box.

Purity Farms
www.purityfarms.com
Organic ghee.

Living Harvest
www.livingharvest.com
(888) 690–3958
Hemp oil.

Essential Living Foods
www.essentiallivingfoods.com
Cacao powder.

Ultimate Superfoods
www.ultimatesuperfoods.com

ORGANIZATIONS AND PROGRAMS

Institute of Integrative Nutrition
www.integrativenutrition.com
This school teaches holistic nutrition that helps integrate mainstream medical philosophy with holistic healing.

The Rose Cleanse
www.detoxworld.com
Natalia Rose teaches about detoxification.

The Cornucopia Institute

www.cornucopia.org/

Seeking economic justice for the family-scale farming community. Through research, advocacy, and economic development, their goal is to empower farmers, partnered with consumers, in support of ecologically produced local, organic, and authentic food.

Veg Source

www.vegsource.com

The Vegan Society

www.vegansociety.com/

Vegan Athlete

www.veganathlete.com

Vegan Fitness Website

www.veganfitness.net

Physicians Committee for Responsible Medicine

www.pcrm.org
5100 Wisconsin Ave. NW, Suite 404
Washington, DC 20016
(202) 686–2210

I joined this before I was a vegetarian and found it to be an amazing source of information on promoting preventative medicine, higher standards of ethics, and effective research. It offers vegetarian starter kits. Dr. Neal Barnard is a part of this organization.

Food and Water

www.foodandwater.org
389 Rt. 215
Walden, VT 05873
(800) EAT–SAFE

This group can provide information on food and water, leading campaigns against toxic and unsafe food and water practices, and helping protect our water.

Association of Veterinarians for Animal Rights

www.avar.org
P.O. Box 208
Davis, CA 95617
(530) 759–8106

This group works on animal protection issues, especially those involving veterinary medical ethics.

People for the Ethical Treatment of Animals (PETA)

www.peta-online.org
501 Front St.
Norfolk, VA 23510
(757) 622–PETA

PETA works to expose inhumane treatment of animals, and helps foster respect and understanding for all creatures and the environment.

Endangered Species Coalition

www.stopextinction.org
1101 14th St. NW, Suite 1400
Washington, DC 20005
(202) 682–9400

Promotes work to protect and recover at-risk species.

Farm Animal Reform Movement (FARM)

www.farmusa.org
P.O. Box 30654
Bethesda, MD 20824
(888) FARM–USA

This group promotes vegetarianism and advocates for the well-being of farm animals.

Farm Sanctuary

www.factoryfarming.com
P.O. Box 150
Watkins Glen, NY 14891
(607) 583–2225
and
P.O. Box 1065
Orland, CA 95963
(530) 865–4617

This group provides refuge for animals rescued from factory farms, stockyards, and slaughterhouses. It operates a bed and breakfast for visitors to the sanctuary.

Food Animal Concerns Trust (FACT)

www.foodanimalconcerns.org
P.O. Box 14599

Chicago, IL 60614
(773) 525–4952

FACT promotes more humane, safe, and sustainable methods of raising livestock and poultry, and runs food safety and on-farm programs.

***Vegetarian Times* Magazine**
www.vegetariantimes.com

Culture and Animals Foundation (CAF)
www.cultureandanimals.org

Founded by Tom and Nancy Regan, CAF is a non-profit organization committed to fostering the growth of intellectual and artistic endeavors united by a positive concern for animals. CAF exists to expand the understanding and appreciation of animals, improving the ways in which they are treated and their standing in society.

PROBIOTIC FOODS

Inner-Eco
www.inner-eco.com
A coconut, power-packed probiotic kefir.

High Country
www.highcountrykombucha.com

Happy Herbalist
www.happyherbalist.com/kombucha.htm
Kombucha-making kits.

Garden of Life
www.gardenoflife.com
Raw kombucha in capsule form.

The Body Ecology (Donna Gates's site)
www.bodyecology.com

This is a good site to visit if you think you have a *Candida* problem and need a resource, and it is a good source of information in general. There are also some great products that you can purchase such as coconut probiotic drinks, recipes, etc. Donna Gates also works in conjunction with doctors and helping children with autism.

SEEDS AND SPROUTING SUPPLIES

The Hippocrates Health Institute

www.hippocrateshealthinstitute.com
1443 Palmdale Court
West Palm Beach, FL 33411

This is a great resource for seeds, equipment, raw food, vegan food, etc., and a great place to go for healthy rejuvenation of the body.

Got Sprouts

www.gotsprouts.com

Seeds of Change

www.seedsofchange.com

This is my favorite place to purchase seeds. They have organic gardening seeds.

This company also makes wonderful, high-quality organic food products.

Probiotics for the Garden, People, and Pets

I use this for cleaning my seeds, feeding my garden, composting, and flea prevention for my pets. (It is used by the SPCA for flea prevention in a natural way.)

TeraGanix, Inc. (formerly EM America)

www.teraganix.com

The exclusive distributor of Dr. Higa's Effective Microorganisms EM•1® Microbial Inoculants in the United States.

SNACK BARS

Raw Crunch Bars

rawcrunchbar.myshopify.com/

These are great for food on the go and come in cranberry, chocolate, goji berry, and blueberry.

Fruits of Life by Garden of Life

www.organichealthylifestyle.com (order from my website)

Their organic raw bars are especially delicious. There are quite a few flavors to choose from. My favorite is chocolate raspberry. The chocolate-covered greens bar with live probiotic is another one of my favorite quick snacks when I don't have time for a meal.

SOAPS AND CLEANING PRODUCTS

Dean Vanderslice
Edits! Interiors

www.editsinteriors.com

Non-toxic cleaning products with essential oils.

Dr. Bronner's Magic Soap

www.drbronner.com

(760) 743–2211

This is a blend of pure castille soap. Some contain essential oils. I buy them in large bottles and use them to refill my hand soap containers.

Oxo Brite

www.ecos.com

This is a great, non-toxic stain remover that I use on almost all my stains. I put a scoop or two in a bowl of water and soak my stained clothing overnight. It really brightens white, too.

Twenty Mule Team Borax

www.20muleteamlaundry.com

One of the best all-purpose cleaners! It is a natural mineral and is so inexpensive. You won't believe how great this is!

SPICES

Frontier Natural Products

www.frontiercoop.com

Mountain Rose Company

www.mountainroseherbs.com/

TEAS

Organic India

www.organicindia.com

A brand of tulsi tea.

Yogi Tea

www.yogiproducts.com

Good selection of organic teas.

Mountain Rose Herbs

www.mountainroseherbs.com/

An amazing selection of rarer teas, herbs, oils, information, etc.

Celestial Seasonings Tea

www.celestialseasonings.com

GT's Kombucha Tea

www.GTSkombucha.com

(877) RE-Juice

Organic, raw kombucha.

VACATION/RETREAT AND SPA DESTINATIONS

Omega

eomega.org

(877) 944–2002 (US)

(845) 266–4444 (international)

E-mail: registration@eomega.org

This woodland retreat in New York state is a wonderful place to visit if you're interested in participating in a holistic workshop or are just looking for a change of environment. Though not luxurious, it is an amazing vacation destination. It offers a large variety of classes, ranging from spiritual and art classes to dance and yoga. I think of it as a camp for adults. Its mission statement is: "Through innovative educational experiences that awaken the best in the human spirit, Omega provides hope and healing for individuals and society." It has a new campus in Costa Rica as well.

Fairmont Hotels

www.fairmont.com/en_fa

This luxury hotel chain boasts over 50 distinctive eco-friendly hotels around the world. Fairmont is working on a Green Partnership. Its restaurants have vegetarian, vegan, gluten-free, and raw meals on the menu.

The Homestead

www.thehomestead.com/

This historic hotel is nestled amid the beautiful Allegheny Mountains. I love to go there for the hot springs. You will feel like you have gone back in time with the elegance of the place. It has wonderful golf courses, skiing in winter, horseback riding, and a wonderful spa.

Ojo Caliente Mineral Springs Resort & Spa

ojospa.com/contact.php

(800) 222–9162

(505) 583–2233

This place is one hour from Santa Fe in Ojo Caliente, New Mexico. This spa is one of the oldest mineral spring spas in the United States. It has four different types of mineral waters (lithium, iron, soda, and arsenic), over 100,000 gallons a day, that still come steaming to the surface, revitalizing those who soak in these legendary waters.

The Get Well Retreat

getwellretreat.com/projects.php

This is a non-profit, community outreach group that holds holistic, wellness retreats at the Deep Bay Retreat Center on Flathead Lake. Its retreats are centered around helping people develop a more holistic lifestyle for the benefit of their physical and spiritual well-being. I highly recommend these retreats for the adventurous souls undaunted by a more rustic facility.

Its mission is:

> "We believe that food is our medicine, exercise is our strength, and knowledge is our power. The majority of our health problems stem from what we eat and how we think. We know we can change this! The retreats are organized by local health care professionals dedicating to bringing wellness to our community. The retreats are fun, relaxing, informative, and motivating. Following the retreat, we have on-going training and support within our communities for wellness coaching, raw food preparation, exercise, and sustainable living, so we can help ourselves and families thrive for the long run."

I have been to a few of these retreats and had a wonderful experience. I plan to return.

The Happy Cow

www.happycow.net/travel/bb_retreats.html

This is a web site where you can look up vegetarian places all over the world. It lists restaurants, bed and breakfasts, hotels, resorts, etc.

VEGAN SUPPLIES OF ALL VARIETIES

Vegan Store

www.veganstore.com

VITAMINS

Buy vitamins made with whole, organic food. The body reads whole food much better than it does isolated chemicals.

Garden of Life

www.organichealthylifestyle.com (order from my website)

I love the organic, raw, whole-food vitamin B complex by Garden of Life.

New Chapter Organics

www.newchapter.com

A variety of whole-food-based and organic products.

Ancient Minerals

www.magneticclay.com

Ultra-pure magnesium oil.

Peter Gillham's Natural Vitality

www.petergillham.com

This is a magnesium powder supplement that can be mixed with water. It has a natural, calm, raspberry-lemon flavor.

Glutamine Powder

www.iron-tek.com

This is an essential Glutamine Powder by Iron Tek.

Food-Grade Hydrogen Peroxide

www.narualzing.com

This Natural Zing hydrogen peroxide is great for cleaning fruits and vegetables.

Sunrider

www.organichealthylifestyle.com (order from my website or contact me)

I often use Sunrider's supplements, teas, and foods. Their quinary supplement, a concentrated, food-grade, herb supplement, especially helped me stop drinking coffee. In addition, their stevia is my favorite brand of stevia.

WINE

Frey Vineyards

www.freywine.com
Redwood Valley, CA 95470
Organic wine without added sulfites.

Benefit Wines

www.benefitwines.com/peta
Vegan-friendly, organic wines.

Appendix A

Recipe Index

Appendix B

Index of Raw Recipes

Appendix C

A Walk Through the Grocery Store

Let me simply walk through the grocery store with you. Here are some ideas for going to the grocery store and what to look for.

Look for labels that say that the food is organic. You want organically grown and produced foods. The label may say "certified organic," meaning that it had the certification issued from the USDA. If it is organic, it was supposed to be grown from seed that was not genetically engineered. (I do see canola oil that is certified organic, and it is a genetically engineered seed. Alas, this is a discrepancy, because the USDA says it doesn't allow genetically engineered seeds to be used.) There are two basic types of genetically engineered crops on the market now: herbicide-tolerant and insect-resistant.

Herbicide-tolerant crops usually include corn, cotton, sugar beets, soy, and canola. These are grown to handle the direct use of pesticides on them. There are over a billion pounds of pesticides used in the United States alone each year. Many of these chemical fertilizers were developed for use as bombs or poisons in warfare. They poison our food and our environment. Pesticides particularly affect our nervous system.

Insect-resistant crops usually include corn, potatoes, soy, and cotton. These plants actually produce an insecticide to kill insects that feed on them. If this is what the genetically engineered plant is doing to a small insect, then what is it doing to the person who is eating this food? The effect of this type of plant on the environment and in the human body, especially long-term, is unknown.

Genetically engineered, or genetically modified (GM), plants are escaping into the wild and inter-breeding with wild plants. Our pollinators, such as bees, are in trouble now. Are genetically engineered plants a contributing factor? Good question. Genetically engineered food is such a recent food product that no long-term, in-depth studies show their long-term effect on humans or the ecosystem. You must decide for yourself if eating food that has pest control built right into it or has large amounts of poisons put on it is good for human consumption.

"An estimated 75 percent of foods in U.S. grocery stores contain GM ingredients. About seven out of every 10 items in the average grocery cart have been genetically modified. And don't bother reading labels to see if you're buying a GM product, because *no labeling is required.*"[165]

Another thing food venders do to make produce more appealing to consumers is to dip it in color or wax, or put a preservative on it produce to make it look prettier. Organic food is supposed to be grown without chemical, synthetic, or biological pest control or fertilizers used. Although the USDA continues to water down its regulations, certified organic is still better than non-certified organic. This is because the USDA organic label gives you the most information about the origins and production of your food. These foods must adhere to much stricter regulations than any other food on the market, and the stricter the regulations, the more you will know about what is actually in your food, thus, giving you more control over what you put into your body and empowering you to make more informed decisions at the grocery store.

You may want to let your voice be heard in favor of stricter food labeling and production regulations. Personally, I would like to see foods containing genetically modified ingredients labeled as such, as is currently required in most Western countries. If you would like to make your voice heard, call your local representatives and senators and let them know how you feel. Join the Organic Consumers Association (www.organicconsumers.org) and keep up with the bills and laws.

Produce

Start by trying to buy fruits and vegetables that are in season. They will be fresher and less expensive. Most fruits and vegetables in our stores are about five days old. They are picked, packed, shipped, and unpacked before we buy them. Look for vibrancy of color, or smoothness, and freshness of skin. Try to buy organic so foods aren't artificially colored, waxed, or dipped to make them look commercially better for market. Smell food for freshness. Look for bruises, cuts, or mold when buying anything fresh, especially if the food is in a plastic container or bag.

Our body needs food that is in season because it works in harmony with the seasons. In-season foods will be a better buy and may even be grown locally. If food is grown locally it is probably fresher. When food is picked, it starts to die. It will still have living enzymes in it, but the enzymes fade as time passes. Therefore, the more recently the food was picked, the more living enzymes it contains. The freshest food is ripened on the vine, and then picked and eaten as soon as possible. Really look at the food you buy. Look for smooth, firm, undamaged produce that smells fresh.

As I mentioned, I highly recommend always buying certified organic food. Support the farmers who are not poisoning the environment, and buy food that is free of pesticides and chemical fertilizers. Children are much more sensitive to these poisons because their organs are still forming.

All pesticides are not created equal. Some are worse than others. The following may help you decide what you should buy non-organic.

Foods with the **highest** use of pesticides:	Foods that usually have the **lowest** use of pesticides:
Apples	Avocados
Bell Peppers	Asparagus
Celery	Bananas
Cherries	Broccoli
Grapes	Cabbage
Lettuce	Corn
Nectarines	Kiwi
Peaches	Mangoes
Pears	Onions
Potatoes	Papaya
Spinach	Peas
Strawberries	Pineapples

Clean all fruits and vegetables before you eat them. Apple cider vinegar works well and isn't very expensive. Use 1 tablespoon for each gallon of water, or ¼ cup for a sink full of water. Let fruits and vegetables soak at least 15 minutes. I clean everything, even things I peel (like avocados) because the knife that cuts through food will pull toxins from the outer skin into the food.

Mushrooms

When the weather is cold, I love something savory and hearty like mushrooms, which are surprisingly rich in nutrients. These dense, smooth, earthy fungi grow in thousands of varieties and have been studied extensively for their health benefits. Studies show that mushrooms aid the immune system because they are rich in anti-oxidants, potassium, selenium, copper, riboflavin, niacin, and pantothenic acid. In addition, select mushrooms are one of only two natural food sources of Vitamin D. One medium portobello mushroom has 407 mg of potassium, compared to a small banana having 362 mg, while an orange has 237 mg and four–five small button mushrooms have 237 mg. Selenium is an important mineral that works as an anti-oxidant to protect the body and support the immune system. Four or five medium cremini mushrooms have 21.8 mcg of selenium, as compared to one large egg with 15 mcg, 3 ounces of lean beef with 18.1 mcg, a portobello mushroom with 9.2 mcg, or four–five white mushrooms with 7.8 mcg. In addition, the copper in mushrooms helps make red blood cells, which carry oxygen throughout the body.

Mushrooms are easy to add to your meals and diet. When you buy them, look for mushrooms that are smooth, clean, and fresh in appearance. Keep them in the same container they come in, and refrigerate them until you're ready to use them. To clean them, use a soft mushroom brush or wet paper towel to remove any parts that look dirty or mushy. You can rinse them, but do not soak them. They can keep up to a week in the refrigerator in a porous paper bag, but never put mushrooms in an airtight container and never freeze them. Also, always trim the end of the stem before you use mushrooms. Many of the stems are too tough, so just use the caps if this is the situation.

There is a huge variety of mushrooms, thousands of which are poisonous, so do *not* pick them in the wild. Always buy them from a reliable and reputable supplier.

Adding mushrooms to dishes is easy. Thinly slice some mushrooms and put them on salads, in pasta dishes, or on sandwiches, or serve them as a side dish. Grilling them is always great, and mushrooms make a good vegetarian alternative to a burger. I love to sauté them with onions and butter to bring out the rich flavor of savory mushrooms. Each mushroom has a different flavor, so experiment and try a different variety every now and then.

Sprouts

When I was editing this book, my editor asked me why this food has its own section. Because this food is so incredibly nutritious and so incredibly power-packed, sprouts simply needed their own section!

Sprouts are the ultimate super-food. Sprouts are the basis of life; they rejuvenate, re-energize, and heal. Sprouts are one of the most complete and nutritionally rich sources of all foods tested for nutrients. Sprouts can contain all the nutritional value of the whole plant in one little sprout! The Chinese have included sprouts as a nutritional part of their diet for thousands of years. The mung bean is one of my favorite sprouts. A sprouted mung bean has the carbohydrate content of a melon, Vitamin A of a lemon, thiamin of an avocado, riboflavin of a dry apple, niacin of a banana, and ascorbic acid of a loganberry—in one sprout! In a newspaper article by Linden Staciokas, Dr. Paul Talalay of the American Cancer Society is quoted as saying that "broccoli sprouts are better for you than full-grown broccoli, and contain more of the enzyme sulforaphane which helps protect cells and prevents their genes from turning into cancer."[166]

Sprouts are a complete food containing protein, carbohydrates, and "good" fat. They are rich in vitamins, minerals, and natural enzymes. Studies have shown that when seeds and grains are germinated they increase in nutrients and enzymes "25 to 4,000 percent."[167] Because of the protein shortage during World War II, Dr. Clive M. McKay promoted sprouted soybeans as a wartime food source.

It is really easy to make your own sprouts. Anyone can do it. All you need are seeds, clean water, and nutrient-rich soil. After about four days the seed is ready to harvest. This is an easy way to add a wealth of nutrition to your food. The FDA said contaminated food plant seeds could cause food-borne illness, so cleaning seeds is recommended. Clean seeds with a mixture of lime juice and vinegar or a tiny bit of food-grade hydrogen peroxide. Later on you will soak them with EM, an effective microbial inoculant or probiotic blend I learned about at a Tree of Life Organic Gardening class. This is because the seeds and the earth benefit from probiotics, boosting their ability to fight off "bad" or harmful bacteria, just as our body benefits from probiotics, which keep "bad bacteria" in check. In a sense, we are boosting the earth's immune system. Microbial inoculant products include three groups of naturally occurring beneficial bacteria: yeast, photosynthetic bacteria, and lactic acid bacteria. The probiotic "works together with microbes in the area to which it is added to promote a healthy environment for beneficial microorganisms and larger forms of life including insects and worms, pets, livestock and people."[168]

So, step one after cleaning the seeds is to soak them in a mild mixture of one drop of EM in 1 cup of pure water and let them sit for about 10 minutes. Then put the seeds in pure, healthy water and soak them overnight. Once the seeds have been soaked overnight, drain the water. Put them in a colander or a sprouting bag or jar, and then put the container you have chosen in a dark, cool place. (The ideal temperature is around 70 degrees.) Keep them in the dark. You can leave them in the colander, sprouting bag, or sprouting jar. (I simply lay a dish towel over my sprouts or put them in a dark room.) Rinse the seeds one to three times a day with pure water, until they start to sprout. When they start to sprout, they will grow quickly. After a full day or two sprouting, you can move them to the sunlight. There they will develop chlorophyll, the green pigment found in plants.

Chlorophyll has anti-inflammatory and anti-oxidant properties. These anti-oxidants prevent or slow down oxidation, which leads to cell damage. Once this oxidation occurs, these newly formed, abnormal cells begin to reproduce. This oxidation can be attributed to aging and most of the diseases associated with living organisms. These anti-oxidants also stop the damage caused by free radicals.

In addition, chlorophyll gives sprouts high levels of oxygen. Nobel Prize–winning Dr. Otto Warburg found that cancer cells, bacteria, and viruses could not survive in a body with high amounts of oxygen.[169] He also found that the body should ideally be around 7 on the pH scale. Processed foods are acidic and can make the body acidic. Sprouts are a great source of oxygen and are also an alkaline food. Leave the sprouts in the sunlight for a day or more to get as much chlorophyll as you can into your sprouts!

Add sprouts to salads, sandwiches, dips, smoothies, green drinks, juices, and more!

Bulk Foods

Some fruits come in packages of four or more. Buying these packages is often more cost-effective than buying them separately. Be sure to check fruit for bruises, cuts, and freshness.

Nuts, seeds, grains, rice, soup mixes, granola, trail mixes, and more can be found in the bulk foods section. These can be less expensive, and there may be more turnover in this area of the store, so the food is often fresher than what is already bagged/packaged. Be certain to read the ingredients completely to see if they have added sugar or any other ingredients you are not expecting, and make sure they have an organic label. Nut butters, maple syrup, honey, and purified water are usually in this section at Whole Foods Market.

Spices, herbs, and tea are great items to buy in bulk. There is a greater turnover in these items as well, and they will probably be fresher than the pre-packaged varieties. Also, you can get the exact amount you need for a dish rather than being left with an entire bottle of a spice or herb you don't use often. Buying bulk spices, herbs, teas, and salts whole and grinding them yourself, or buying them ground in small amounts as needed, is a good practice and likely gives you a fresher product. Store fresh spices, herbs, and teas in airtight glass containers so they keep longer and stay fresher.

Read the Ingredients

Know what is in the food and body products that you buy. The front label of a product can be very misleading. I learned a long time ago that "natural" means nothing. Foods can be completely chemically derived and still say "natural" on the advertisement or package. The US Code of Federal Regulations says a natural flavor or flavoring is

> the essential oil, oleoresin, essence or extractive, protein hydrolysate, distillate, or any product of roasting, heating or enzymolysis, which contains the flavoring constituents derived from a spice, fruit or fruit juice, vegetable or vegetable juice, edible yeast, herb, bark, bud, root, leaf or similar plant material, meat, seafood, poultry, eggs, dairy products, or fermentation products thereof, whose significant function in food is flavoring rather than nutritional.[170]

In the book *Fast Food Nation*, Eric Schlosser says,

> Consumers prefer to see natural flavors on a label,

> out of a belief that they are healthier. The distinction between artificial and natural flavors can be arbitrary and somewhat absurd, based more on how the flavor has been made than on what it actually contains.[171]

He goes on to say:

> A natural flavor is not necessarily healthier or purer than an artificial one. When almond flavor (benzaldehyde) is derived from natural sources, such as peach and apricot pits, it contains traces of hydrogen cyanide, a deadly poison.[172]

A product may say olive oil is in the product, but the ingredients may list canola oil or something else as well, or a larger amount than what was advertised on the packaging. Shop prepared: Take your reading glasses with you, because ingredients are printed so small sometimes that they can be very difficult to read. Foods like bread, crackers, and pasta can also be very misleading. Read ingredient lists carefully. Look for chemicals and additives.

Take pasta, for example. Pasta is product that you should always buy as a whole grain. Read the label and make certain that it says "whole grain" and that it has the same ingredients that the packaging indicates it has. There are some really good whole-grain pastas, some of which are even gluten-free, like quinoa, spelt, and rice pasta. Quinoa is also a complete protein, so it is a good choice for vegetarians or vegans. Sprouted grains are also more digestible, so look for any kind of sprouted grains in breads, crackers, cereals, etc.

Raw food sometimes contains a great deal of sugar, so always check the amount. I try not to buy foods with agave nectar, canola oil, or non-whole-grain flour. And remember that "natural" means nothing in labeling. Companies also use the term "natural" as an alias for adding MSG to food. Be aware of this and look for natural flavorings, coloring, and so forth on ingredient lists. If in doubt, ask a store employee for more information about a product. Whole Foods employees, for example, often go out of their way to help with any questions or concerns you may have about their various products.

Read labels carefully. Products marked "low-fat" or "fat-free" are usually less healthy than the full-fat versions. This is just a marketing gimmick. Many of these products have added sugar or white refined salt, and may actually have chemicals in them.

Beware of the power of advertising; it can lead you to believe you are buying one thing when you are really being sold something else. Packaging is big business, and it can be misleading. Be a smart and savvy shopper.

Packaging

Most cans are lined with BPA, which is a synthetic estrogen and hormone disruptor. BPA-free packaging can be found. Look for BPA-free packaging or the numbers on plastic packaging, which will indicate if it is safe. Safe plastic packages will be numbered 1, 2, 4, 5, and 6. When all is said and done, however, glass is always the safest option.

Baking Section

This section of the store should have extra-virgin olive oil, extra-virgin, pure coconut oil, ghee, apple cider vinegar, Celtic sea salt, spices, yeast, various types of flours and sugars, other oils, parchment paper, and baking needs.

Asian Foods

This area of the store should contain different types of soy sauces, miso, plum paste, and seaweed varieties. Freeze-dried soups and foods are good to pack for travel emergency meals, emergency meals for home, or camping. These don't usually require a can opener and can be used in many situations with only a little water added to hydrate them.

Snack Food Bars, Chocolate Bars, Protein Bars, and Raw Food Bars

Read labels. Make sure what is advertised is what is listed in the ingredients! Whey is a dairy. I do not recommend this as a food bar ingredient. Many good food bars that are raw, organic, and made with whole foods and/or protein (made up of sprouted grains, nuts, seeds, and other ingredients) do not contain whey or soy. Check the sugar and salt content. Many contain agave nectar, which can have an even higher glycemic index than high-fructose corn syrup. Be aware of this if you have high blood sugar.

Coconut water is usually on the shelves in this area with the health food bars or "raw" food bars. Coconut water is rich in electrolytes. It was used in many wars as a substitute for blood when blood was needed but unavailable for blood transfusions. Coconut water shares many of the same properties as human blood. It is extremely hydrating and rich in nutrients. It is a great post-workout drink or water alternative.

Super-Foods and/or Raw Foods

Super-foods are foods that have more nutrients in them than many "normal," everyday foods. Raw, vegan, gluten-free super-foods are usually in an area all by themselves. You can find meal-replacement protein powder that is raw, vegan, organic, and gluten-free, green concentrated powders, chia seeds, cacao powder, goji berries (wolf berries), acai berries, golden berries, and maca root.

Frozen Foods

Stores usually offer some choices for breads, imitation meats, easy meals, healthy ice creams, and frozen fruits and vegetables. Most growers who freeze their produce do so within hours of the produce being picked, so frozen foods may be more nutrient-dense than some fresh foods. Frozen fruits are good in smoothies, and they make smoothies colder without getting watery from adding ice. Some raw food practitioners think that freezing food changes it molecularly. Many raw food people don't eat or buy frozen foods. Decide what works for you, and live your life accordingly.

Breads, Crackers, and Chips

Have you ever been in the bread or cracker aisle at the supermarket, with all the choices of "all natural," "whole wheat," "whole grain," "sprouted," and "organic"? These are some words that have become really attractive to us, especially if we are trying to buy the healthiest foods. These words on food packaging can be misleading, though.

By labeling standards, products are required to use only a small percentage of whole-grain ingredients in order to list "whole grain" on their label. A product can be mostly white, refined flour and still have "whole grain" or "whole wheat" on the label, as long as there's some whole grain or whole wheat in it. Look to see that "100% whole organic grain" or "100% whole wheat" is the very first ingredient listed, so you are not tricked into buying a product made of mostly white, refined wheat, or other flour that has had the nutrition-rich part of the grain removed.

(Ingredients are listed in order of the amount used in the product.) Most of the nutrients are in the germ of the grain, and the hull is the fiber. When these are removed (as is the case with white flour), the grain is left devoid of nutrients or fiber, and the body reads this as sugar.

The first four to five ingredients are really important, because they make up the bulk of a product. Wheat has a unique ability to raise blood sugar extremely quickly.

Blue corn has 20% more protein, 8% less starch, and a lower glycemic index than yellow corn. If you are buying chips or tortillas, look for the blue variety.

"Sprouted" is another term seen in food products today. When a grain is sprouted, it makes the grain much more digestible. Many bread, cracker, and cereal products today have sprouted grains listed on the package or in the ingredient list. Look for the words "sprouted whole grain" in the list of ingredients.

Our thyroid is our master gland. It is central to all of our body's major functions. It influences our metabolism, digestion, energy, body temperature, skin, hair, sleep, mental acuity, nervous system, sexual organs, and hormonal system. In fact, it would be very difficult to find a system that is *not* influenced by the thyroid. The main nutrient that supports our thyroid is iodine. Up until 1980, bakeries added iodine to bread. After that they switched to potassium bromate.

What does this mean? We have a certain amount of space for the iodine in our thyroid. When we ingest potassium bromate, it acts like iodine. It will take up the space for iodine and actually prevent your body from absorbing the iodine it needs. This contributes to iodine deficiency. Check ingredient lists or ask at the bakery if potassium bromate is put in the bakery goods.

According to the Center for Science and Public Interest (CSPI), the FDA has known that bromate causes cancers in laboratory animals, but has failed to ban it. Canada banned it in 1994 and Great Britain in 1990.[173] "The FDA should fulfill its responsibility to protect the public's health," said Michael F. Jacobson, PhD, executive director of CSPI.[174] Instead of meeting privately with the potassium bromate industry, the FDA should ban bromate immediately. When the FDA tested foods in 1992–1993 and again in 1998–1999, many baked goods contained unsafe levels of potassium bromate.

Check packages of Pepperidge Farm, Pillsbury, and Best Foods, Inc. (maker of Arnold, Entenmann's, and Oroweat brands) products. They say they have switched to bromate-free processes. Make sure you read the ingredient list of bakery goods for this ingredient.

Grains

Buy grains, rice, and beans in the freshest, most whole form that you can. The nutrients are in the germ, right below the hull. The hull is the fiber, and the germ is the nutritious part. So, for the most nutritious food, buy whole grains in all of the choices of grains and rice. This is one of the best ways to get protein. Grains are inexpensive and delicious, and there is a huge variety. Try to buy organic. When ready to use, rinse grains. Grains have been milled and stored in storage units or silos (probably in a place where bugs, mice, rats, and snakes can be found). I use a fine, mesh colander to rinse grains.

Organic, Local Milk, Cheese, and Eggs

One weekend I went to some local organic farms just outside of Dallas. I wanted to see for myself if what I had been told at the farmer's market was really true. I was so amazed at the information I learned on this adventure. Some of these farms are completely organic, but not certified. It costs another five or six thousand dollars to get certified, and some farmers don't produce enough to make it worth their effort and money to do that. Other farms I visited did have the certification.

Some farms I visited raised goats (for fresh, raw goat milk), chickens (for eggs), and/or cows for dairy. These farms were impressive. They were incredibly healthy and well managed. Some of them pumped water from their clean pond (never used by the animals for bathing) to the animals' drinking troughs. All of the animals were out in a large green pastures with shade trees and room to roam and play.

These farmers taught me a lot about certain types of labeling. Farmers use many different labels on packages of eggs, poultry, and milk products. Chickens in large farming practices can be called free-range if they have "access" to a place where they can move around, even if that's a cement room that they never even get to go into. Chickens can be called cage-free if they are not in cages. Cage-free can mean a huge, overcrowded room of chickens that can barely move. Free-roaming means they have 18 inches of dirt; it does not mean grass, fresh air, or sunlight. I have found some local farmers who raise chickens in green pastures with spring water, fresh air, and sunlight. The chickens have houses they are able to go into, nest, and produce eggs. When I buy my eggs, I buy them at the farmer's market from these farmers. These eggs are usually a day or two old. (Since they are so fresh, they may have a different color than the ones you are used to buying at the store.)

The cows at this farm are 100% grass-fed. I learned that more antacids are used on cattle in feed lots and factory farms than on humans. Cows that eat what I call "not normal" food ("normal" being grasses and green vegetation from the land) have trouble digesting grains and seed oils (which I call "not normal") and therefore have terrible stomach acid. Animals that are fed organic food aren't necessarily fed the natural food these animals would normally eat in the wild. They can be organically raised animals, but not be eating properly for their species, which affects the animals. Stress breaks down the immune system, so stressed animals will have a weakened immune system.

This farmer moves animals from pasture to pasture without rough cowboys and in a calm and loving way, in order for the land to rest and acquire the nutrients from manure the animals leave on the pastures and without stressing the animals. This farmer lets each pasture rest two to four months before putting the animals back. This allows the grasses to grow back with the nutrients of the composted manure. The soil was very healthy, as seen by the worm castings everywhere I walked. (Worms thrive in healthy soil.)

Grass-fed cows can be fed grain and are often fed grain and/or seed oil (like cotton seed oil) to fatten them. Animals suffer and consumers suffer because of these practices. These practices affect the milk and cheese. Find a 100% grass-fed cow. I like raw milk and cheese that has not been pasteurized. This means it has the live enzymes and probiotics in a greater quantity than in the pasteurized versions. Find cheese with vegetarian enzymes, not animal rennet. Goat milk and cheese are more digestible for humans than cow milk.

Most cities have some farms in the area that grow food and raise animals in an organically sound way. One thing you can do to find out about these farms is to find groups that support organic, fresh, slow foods and see if there is a co-op for organic food in the area. You can go to meet-ups or co-ops online in your area and find a group. (One link to check out is www.localharvest.org.) The next time you are in the supermarket and see cheaply priced eggs, milk, and cheese, think about why it looks so good for being so cheap. When you buy from a small farmer with organic, healthy, environmentally friendly farming practices, you are voting with your pocketbook for these farmers to survive and thrive.

One thing you might want to think about is that drinking milk from another animal is really not natural. Cows and goats only give milk when they need to feed their babies. A baby cow weighs about 75 to 100 pounds and needs to become 2,000 pounds in about two years. This is a lot of weight to gain. Farmers have to keep cows or goats pregnant in order for the animals to continue making milk. This is something else to consider.

Many of us, when making food choice transitions, may need to make baby steps toward new food choices. Vegan and alternative milks and cheeses are really delicious, but they do taste a little different. Try tasting a few and adding them to your diet a little at a time. I added non-dairy milks to my milk a little each time I had it. I added more each time, and I eventually switched. That process worked for me.

Vegan, raw food nut cheeses are delicious. Give them a try and let your taste buds start to change in that direction. We develop new taste buds on a continual basis. If you want to "learn" to like something, start trying it daily or regularly (at least 10 times or for two weeks). You will find that your taste buds will adjust.

Dairy is hard for many people to digest. When mammals are born, they have a lactase enzyme to help digest their mother's milk. By about age 4, mammals lose most of that enzyme, so digesting milk is much harder. Also, milk products that are pasteurized are acidic in nature, and our pH balance is very important to maintain health. The dairy industry advertises calcium in milk, but if it is acidic, our body can pull calcium from the bones in order to adjust the pH balance from all the acidic dairy being consumed.[175]

If you are worried about iron, dairy is not a good thing to consume. A study reported in the *American Journal of Clinical Nutrition* in 1987 said that the calcium from dairy products impairs absorption of iron and blocks its transport across the cells lining in the small intestines.[176] In the book *Fit For Life II,* Harvey and Marilyn Diamond say, "Dairy Products ARE DIS-EASE PRODUCING."[177]

Think about finding some alternatives to dairy in your diet. I put one of my clients on a dairy-free diet and she did not think she could do it.

Within one week, she said she had no more acid reflux disease and was sleeping all night for the first time in a very long time. I have included some recipes that include cheese products in this book. I recommend using goat milk cheese, because it is more easily digested than cow milk. I also recommend using organic, raw, unpasteurized milk products from a reliable organic source—a facility and animals in extremely healthful environments with fresh air, sunshine, exercise, and healthy, natural food. There are some really good raw cheese vegan cheese recipes in Alissa Cohen's living food books (*Living on Live Food* and *Raw Food for Everyone*).

As for eggs, I only buy my eggs from a farmer who raises his chickens in a healthy, grass, fresh-air, fresh-water, no-abuse environment, where the chickens eat organic, healthy, natural chicken food. The egg industry is not kind to chickens who don't lay or aren't laying anymore. "Organic" does not mean the animal is treated kindly or fairly. As I said, labeling is misleading. If you want to use eggs, I highly recommend finding a local farmer who is kind and thoughtful about how his chickens are raised, treated, and handled. The quality of the food will be much better, and so will your peace of mind.

Cheese and Jelled Food

When I first became vegetarian, I didn't realize animals' stomach substances are put in cheese to make it firm. It is called rennet. This is a meat product. I now look for cheese that has vegetarian ingredients in it. Sometimes it is fig, but many times the product will just say something like "vegetable enzymes."

Gelatin capsules are also meat-based. Gelatin is taken from the hooves or nails and hair of animals. Look for vegetarian capsules made with things like agar. Agar is a seaweed extract that can be used instead of gelatin, and you can substitute it for gelatin in recipes most of the time. It does need to be heated in order to dissolve. It needs to be dissolved slowly and with continual stirring.

When making a Jell-O type of fruit dish, use agar flakes. Heat them slowly while stirring constantly. The flakes will dissolve from the middle toward the outside of the mixture. Mix this dissolved agar flakes mixture with fruit juices for a nice jelled dish.

Appendix D

Basic Kitchen Equipment

1. **Blender.** A blender is probably my most useful kitchen tool. I use it almost every day. Vitamix is a good brand and has a seven-year warranty, but it costs more than most blenders. I am really hard on my blenders, and I use them almost every day. I was wearing out a blender about every three months. Then I bought my Vitamix. I love it. Mine is over 10 years old now and still working great. Breville and the KTec Champ HP3 blenders are both good as well. With a normal blender, soak hard foods in water overnight to soften them so they won't be so hard on your blender.
2. **Toaster/toaster oven.**
3. **Juicer.** The Breville juicer is pretty easy to use and reliable. I juice carrots and a cucumber almost every day. You cannot juice wheatgrass or sprouts in this type of blender. I tried the Green Star brand, but it wore out fairly quickly with a good deal of use with large vegetables. The Hurom juicer does the same thing as the Green Star. One of my friends has the Hurom juicer and says it works great. She loves her Hurom juicer.
4. **Food processor.** Food processors are very useful for making large amounts of raw food or mixing dense or heavy foods, like hummus. Small ones work just fine for most jobs. If I was buying a large one, I would only buy a 10-inch one. My 12-inch has a gap that, in my opinion, doesn't work as well.
5. **Paring knife and/or large cutting knife.**
6. **Cutting board.** Buy a cutting board that is dishwasher-safe so that it can be really sanitized completely.
7. **Stainless-steel sieve.**
8. **Spatula and scraper.**
9. **Glass, stainless steel, or lead-free ceramic baking dishes.** Be careful about Pyrex dishes. The company was bought by a Chinese company that changed the formula, and now some of the glass cookware has been exploding in heated ovens.[178] I look for antique Pyrex at antique stores and estate sales, where you can

find some really great kitchen equipment for a good price. Aluminum cookware can leach aluminum into the food. Aluminum is linked to Alzheimer's disease.[179] I do not use non-stick cookware. Studies show it releases toxins into the air when heated to high temperatures. "There's a whole chemistry set of compounds that will come off when Teflon is heated high enough to decompose," says Robert L. Wolke, PhD, a professor emeritus of chemistry at the University of Pittsburgh. "Many of these are fluorine-containing compounds, which as a class are generally toxic."[180] "At temperatures above 500°F, the breakdown begins and smaller chemical fragments are released," explains Kurunthachalam Kannan, PhD, an environmental toxicologist at the New York State Department of Health's Wadsworth Center.[181]

Appendix E

Pantry Basics: Foods to Keep on Hand

Sea Salt

Use solar-dried, organic sea salt. This is essential for its minerals. Good-quality, unrefined salt will have about 65 trace minerals. Sea salt is good for you, and will make the flavor of your food more vibrant and tasteful. Salt is a very grounding and can strengthen different parts of the body. It has an alkalizing effect on the body. Natural sea salt is not the same as the processed, bleached brands of salt. It won't have iodine in it, so take an iodine supplement unless you eat a great deal of seaweed.

Sweeteners

- *Stevia:* This is a sweet plant that has no calories. I like the liquid ones best. You just need a drop or two in place of each teaspoon of sugar. Stevia is a good choice for diabetics and/or anyone who wants a healthy, sweet flavor. The Sweet Leaf brand comes in flavors (vanilla, toffee, orange, etc.). I use it to sweeten my tea, nut milks, smoothies, and more.
- *Honey:* Natural, raw honey has antibacterial and anti-toxic properties. It has been used for centuries for burns, sore throats, and stomach disorders.
- *Raw, unrefined sugar:* This is like regular white refined sugar, but it hasn't had all of the nutrients removed. It gives food a richer flavor than white refined sugars.
- *Maple syrup:* This is boiled down from maple tree sap, and is light and sweet.

Black Pepper

Buy whole, raw peppercorns and use a pepper grinder.

Vinegar

Buy raw, unrefined vinegar. (In order for the body to process distilled vinegar, it causes the body to pull minerals from the body, so, I don't recommend buying distilled vinegar to be used in the making of food.) I really like raw, unrefined, organic apple cider vinegar. It is antiparasitic, is anti-fungal, neutralizes poisons, helps with blood circulation, and more. Balsamic vinegar is great to keep in the pantry for making salad dressings or as a dip or spread to use with bread.

Tea

The best teas, in my opinion, are unprocessed and organic. Tea can be used for calming and refreshing the body. Tea can also be used medicinally and ceremoniously.

Spices

I use cinnamon, thyme, parsley, and turmeric frequently. Buy spices in small quantities so that you know they are fresh.

Coconut Oil

Raw, unprocessed, organic, extra-virgin, pure coconut oil is a great choice for all recipes that call for oil.

Extra-Virgin Olive Oil

Buy organic, extra-virgin olive oil in dark glass bottles.

Appendix F

Household Cleaning Products

All of these products are safe, non-toxic, and not tested on animals, and can save you money.

Borax Powder

Twenty Mule Team borax powder is a terrific cleaner! I use it for just about everything: scouring sinks, cleaning windows, cleaning counters, washing floors, laundry boosting, as a dishwashing machine booster, as a refrigerator cleaner, and removing stuck or burned-on food to pots and pans. It is a natural mineral and is only about $3 a box at my grocery store.

White Vinegar

White vinegar kills more germs than bleach. It is also great for removing mildew, stains, and grease. White vinegar also whitens laundry. White vinegar can also be inexpensive. I use it (along with borax powder) for so many of my cleaning needs.

Hydrogen Peroxide

There are two hydrogen peroxide products that I know about. One is the type of hydrogen peroxide that you can buy at the pharmacy and the other is food-grade hydrogen peroxide. Food-grade hydrogen peroxide is very strong and needs to be used with caution, and it needs to be stored in the refrigerator after opening. A study was conducted at Virginia Tech on cleaners that kill germs.[182] Hydrogen peroxide in conjunction with vinegar was found to be the most effective, best germ-killing combination. Hydrogen peroxide and vinegar were put in separate spray bottles, and then used separately but together during the same cleaning. One was sprayed (the vinegar or peroxide; it didn't matter which went first), then the other, and then the surface was wiped clean. Hydrogen peroxide is also inexpensive and non-toxic. How can you beat that?!

All-Purpose Window Cleaner

Combine ¼ cup white vinegar and 1 quart water for a homemade window cleaner. Wear rubber gloves when you are using this, as it can be a little hard on your skin.

Stopped-Up Sinks

Use white vinegar and baking soda to clean and/or to loosen a clogged sink drain.

Furniture Polish

Combine 1 teaspoon lemon oil and about 1 cup coconut or olive oil.

Silver Cleaner

Put at least a 6-inch sheet of aluminum foil in a sink of hot water with at least a tablespoon of baking soda and about a tablespoon of salt. There will be a natural reaction, and the tarnish will disappear from the silver and appear on the foil. This is fun for children to do as a science experiment. You don't even have to scrub or rub. (If you do want to rub, use toothpaste to clean silver.)

Copper, Brass, or Pewter Cleaner

I learned this trick in a gourmet cooking class! Take some salt and some vinegar, and swish it around or rub lightly. There is a chemical reaction, and it cleans the copper. I do this in my copper bowl before I beat my egg whites for soufflés. It makes the egg whites beat quicker and become stiffer quicker.

References

Adams, Mike. "CDC Adjusts Fluoride Poisoning of America's Water Supply to a Lower Level." Natural News website. www.naturalnews.com/030952_CDC_fluoride.html.

——. "Cities Fluoridating Drinking Water with Toxic Chemicals." NewsTarget.com website. March 31, 2005. www.newstarget.com/005900.htm.

"Agriculture Fact Book 98." US Department of Agriculture website. www.usda.gov/news/pubs/fbook98/ch1a.htm.

"Alert: Protein Drinks: You Don't Need the Extra Protein or the Heavy Metals Our Tests Found." *Consumer Reports* website. www.consumerreports.org/cro/magazine-archive/2010/july/food/protein-drinks/overview/index.htm.

Anderson, ND, NMD, Dr. Richard. *Cleanse and Purify Thyself Volume 1, Revised Edition* (Avery Trade, 1991).

——. *Cleanse and Purify Thyself Volume 2, Revised Edition* (Avery Trade, 1998).

Antoniou, Michael, Paul Brack, Andrés Carrasco, John Fagan, and Mohamed Habib. "GM Soy. Sustainable? Responsible?" GMWatch website. www.gmwatch.org/files/GMsoy_Sust_Respons_SUMMARY_ENG_v6.pdf.

"The Arbor, Alcohol and Drug and Rehab." Detox.net website. www.detox.net.au/articles/detoxification.html.

"Average Mineral Content in Selected Vegetables, 1914–1997." Nutrition Security Institute website. www.nutritionsecurity.org/PDF/Mineral%20Content%20in%20Vegetables.pdf.

Azulay, Sol. International Specialty Supply website. www.sproutnet.com/sprouts_in_the_press.htm.

——."There's More to Sprouts than Just a Little Crunch in Your Salad." Interview with the *San Diego Earth Times*. November 1997.

Barclay, Eliza. "What's Best for Kids: Bottled Water or Fountains?" *National Geographic News*, March 3, 2010.

Barnard, MD, Neal. *Food for Life* (Three Rivers Press, 1994).

Barron, Jon. "Myth or Fact: Is Canola Oil Healthy?" Baseline of Health Foundation website. October 9, 2006. www.jonbarron.org/heart-health/bl061009/is-canola-oil-healthy.

Bassler, Dr. Anthony. "A Common Mistake that Prevents Most People from Losing Weight…and How to Avoid It! Why This Simple 'First Step' Should Be Part of Any Weight Management, Anti-Aging and Health Improvement Program." *Vegetarian Times,* January 2004.

Batmanghelidj, Dr. Fereydoon. *ABC of Asthma, Allergies and Lupus, First Edition* (Global Health Solutions, Inc., 2000).

——. *Water: For Health, for Healing, for Life: You're Not Sick, You're Thirsty!* (Hachette Digital, Inc., 2003).

——. *Your Body's Many Cries for Water, Third Edition* (Global Health Solutions, Inc., 2008).

Bellatti, Andy. "You Ask, I Answer: Soy Protein Isolate." Medpedia website. www.medpedia.com/news_analysis/98-Small-Bites/entries/71677-You-Ask-I-Answer-Soy-Protein-Isolate.

Blaylock, R.L. *Excitotoxins: The Taste that Kills* (Health Press, 1994).

Bolen, Jim. "Histamine/Anti-histamine and the Dangers of Taking Anti-histamine." Water Cure website. www.watercure2.org/histamines.htm.

"Bottled Water: Pure Drink or Pure Hype?" Natural Resources Defense Council website. www.nrdc.org/water/drinking/bw/bwinx.asp.

"A Brief History of Protein, Passion, Social Bigotry, Rats and Enlightenment." *The McDougall Newsletter, Volume 2, Number 12,* December 2003. www.nealhendrickson.com/mcdougall/031200puprotein.htm.

Brock, Dr. Rovenia. Interview with Bob Green on foods that help relieve stress. Oprah Radio. January 1, 2008.

Burry, John N. "More on Preventing Skin Cancer: Author's Reply." *British Medical Journal,* November 23, 2003. www.bmj.com/content/327/7425/1228.1.full.

Campbell, T. Colin. "Principles of Nutritional Health. Plant-Based Nutrition." eCornell University and the T. Colin Campbell Foundation. 2010.

Chaitow, Leon. "Candida Albicans: Could Yeast Be Your Problem?" *Harvard Gazette* website. www.news.harvard.edu/gazette/1997/10.30/GeneticSecretso.html.

"Chemicals in the Environment: Chlorine (CAS NO. 7782-50-5)." Prepared by the Office of Pollution Prevention and Toxics. US

Environmental Protection Agency. August 1994.

Cheung, FRCP, Dr. Anthony. "Enzymes." Enerex website. www.enerex.ca/en/articles/digestive-enzymes.

"The 'Chlorinated' Water Issue and the Water Ionization Alternative Using Copper or Silver Nanocrystal Ionization." Biophysica, Inc. website. www.biophysica.com/chlorine.html.

Ciarallo, L., D. Brousseau, and S. Reinert. "Higher-Dose Intravenous Magnesium Therapy for Children with Moderate to Severe Acute Asthma." *Archives of Pediatric & Adolescent Medicine*, October 2000, 154(10): 979–983. National Center for Biotechnology Information website. www.ncbi.nlm.nih.gov/corehtml/pmc/pmcgifs/pmc3_logo_v5.gif.

Coates, Dr. Wayne. "Chia History." Dr. Wayne Coates's website. www.azchia.com/chia_history.htm.

"Code of Federal Regulations, Title 21, Volume 2." Revised as of April 1, 2009. US Government Printing Office. GPO Access CITE: 21CFR101.22. Pages 72–76.

Cohen, Bryan. "Natural Cures for Enlarged Thyroid." eHow website. www.ehow.com/way_5317305_natural-cures-enlarged-thyroid.html#ixzz1SYtyAarn.

Connett, PhD, Paul. "50 Reasons to Oppose Fluoridation." Canton, N.Y.: St. Lawrence University. Food Consumer website. www.foodconsumer.org/newsite/Non-food/Environment/50_reasons_to_oppose_fluoridation_0109111037.html.

"Consumer Group Calls for Ban on 'Flour Improver': Potassium Bromate Termed a Cancer Threat." Center for Science in the Public Interest website. www.cspinet.org/new/bromate.html.

Cousens, MD, Gabriel. *There Is a Cure for Diabetes* (Berkeley, Calif.: North Atlantic Books, 2008).

Cromie, William. "Genetic Secrets of Killer Fungus Found." *Harvard Gazette*, October 30, 1997. news.harvard.edu/gazette/1997/10.30/GeneticSecretso.html.

D'Adamo, Dr. Peter J., with Catherine Whitney. *Eat Right 4 Your Type.* "Blood Type O, Food, Beverage and Supplement List" (Berkley

Books, 1999).

Damato, PhD, Gregory. "GM-Soy: Destroy the Earth and Humans for Profit." Natural News website. May 27, 2009. www.naturalnews.com/026334_soy_Roundup_GMO.html#ixzz1RzIZAWwh.

Dexter, Beatrice. "Honey and Cinnamon: Mother Nature's Powerful Healing Combination." *Weekly World News*, January 17, 1995. weeklyworldnews.com/archive/.

Diamond, Harvey, and Marilyn Diamond. *Fit for Life II* (The Media Business Publishing, 1985).

"Dietary Supplement Fact Sheet: Calcium." US Office of Diet Supplements, National Institutes of Health website. ods.od.nih.gov/factsheets/Calcium-QuickFacts/.

"Dietary Supplement Fact Sheet: Iron." US Office of Dietary Supplements, National Institutes of Health website. ods.od.nih.gov/factsheets/iron/.

"Doing it on Your Own: Eating Vegetarian." McGill University website. June 30, 2010. www.mcgill.ca/fitatmcgill/nutrition/doingit/veg/.

Douillard, DC, Dr. John. "Sun Exposure: Don't Be Fooled By Your Sunscreen." Dr. John Douillard's Lifespa.com website. www.lifespa.com/article.aspx?art_id=114&view=print.

——. "Vitamin D: Astonishing Health Benefits." Dr. John Douillard's Lifespa.com website. www.lifespa.com/article.aspx?art_id=100&view=print.

Downing, MB, BS, Dr. Damien. *Daylight Robbery: The Importance of Sunlight to Health* (Arrow Books, 1998).

Dyer, MS, RD, Diana. "What's in Kale? USDA Nutrient Content Data." 365 Days of Kale weblog. February 22, 2009. www.365daysofkale.com/2009/02/whats-in-kale-usda-nutrient-content.html.

Edwards, Michael. "Healthy Sugar Alternatives: Understanding Both Healthy & Not So Healthy Sugars with Their Glycemic Index." *Organic Lifestyle* magazine, June 12, 2009.

"Eighty Year Decline in Mineral Content of Medium Apple." Nutrition Security Institute website. www.nutritionsecurity.org/PDF/Mineral%20Content%20of%20One%20Apple.pdf.

El, Dr. Akilah M. "The Health Benefits of Bentonite Clay." Dr. Akilah's website: The Natural Health and Holistic World According to Dr. Akilah El. docakilah.wordpress.com/2011/06/09/the-health-benefits-of-bentonite-clay/.

Erasmus, Udo. *Fats That Heal Fats That Kill* (1998).

Fallon, Sally, and Mary G. Enig. "Newest Research on Why You Should Avoid Soy." *Nexus magazine, Volume 7, Number 3,* April–May 2000. www.eregimens.com/therapies/Diet/Soy/NewestResearchonwhyYouShouldAvoidSoy.htm.

Fife, ND, Bruce. *Coconut Cures* (Colorado Springs, Colo.: Piccadilly Books, Ltd., 1952).

"Food from the Rainforests." Rainforest Action Network website. ran.org/fileadmin/materials/education/factsheets/RAN_RainforestFood.pdf.

Francione, Gary, and Robert Garner. *The Animal Rights Debate: Abolition or Regulation* (Columbia University Press, 2010).

Freedman, Rory, and Kim Barnouin. *Skinny Bitch* (Running Press, 2005).

"From the History of Medicine in the USSR." w3.gorge.net/chriss/kombucha.htm.

Gare, Fran. *The Sweet Miracle of Xylitol* (Basic Health Publications, Inc., 2003).

Garland, Cedric F. "Sun Avoidance Will Increase Incidence of Cancers Overall." *British Medical Journal* website. www.bmj.com/content/327/7425/1228.2.full.

Gittleman, PhD, CNS, Ann Louise. *Get the Sugar Out* (New York: Three Rivers Press, 1996).

Gordon, Dennis. "Vegetable Proteins Can Stand Alone." *Journal of the American Dietetic Association, volume 96, issue 3,* March 1996.

Goulart, Frances Sheridan. "Are You Sugar Smart? Linked to Heart Attacks, Kidney Disease, Diabetes and Other Diseases, Sugar Is to the '90s What Cholesterol Was to the '80s—Includes 9 ways to Cope with Sugar Cravings." *American Fitness,* March–April 1991.

Groves, Barry. "Full-Spectrum Sunlight and Cancer: UV Benefits Leukemia and Other Cancers." Second Opinions website. www.

second-opinions.co.uk/full_spectrum_sunlight.html.

Guy, RA. "The Diets of Nursing Mothers and Young Children in Peiping" *Chinese Medical Journal,* 1936; 50:434—442.

Haas, Dr. Elson M., with Dr. Buck Levin. *Staying Healthy with Nutrition* (Celestial Arts, 2006).

Hallberg, Leif, Lena Rossander, and Ann-Britt Skanberg. "Phytates and the Inhibitory Effect of Bran on Iron Absorption in Man." *American Journal of Clinical Nutrition, Volume 45,* 1987: 988–996.

Hattersley, Joseph G. "Poisoning by Chlorinated Water." Dr. Joseph Mercola's website. May 1999. articles.mercola.com/sites/articles/archive/2001/01/07/chlorinated-water2.aspx.

"'Healing Clays' Hold Promise in Fight Against MRSA Superbug Infections and Disease." Arizona State University—Biodesign Institute website. April 7, 2008. www.biodesign.asu.edu.

"High-Fructose Corn Syrup: Everything You Wanted to Know, but Were Afraid to Ask." *American Journal of Clinical Nutrition,* December 2008, 88(6):1715S.

Hooper, Rowan. "Top 11 Compounds in US Drinking Water." *New Scientist,* January 12, 2009. www.newscientist.com/article/dn16397-top-11-compounds-in-us-drinking-water.html.

Howell, Dr. Edward. *Enzyme Nutrition* (Avery Publishing Group Inc., 1985).

——. *Food Enzymes for Health and Longevity* (Omangod Press, 1980), page xiii.

——. *Intestinal Absorption and Secretion.* E. Skadhange, editor (MTP Press Limited, 1984).

——. *Food Enzymes for Health and Longevity, 2nd Edition* (Lotus Press, 1994). Originally published in 1946 as *The Status of Food Enzymes in Digestive and Metabolism.*

"Hunger." FAO news release. September 14, 2010. World Food Programme website. www.wfp.org/hunger/stats,%20FAO%20news%20release,%2014%20September%202010%20%20source.

Hurrell, Richard, Marcel-A Juillerat, Manju Reddy, Sean Lynch, Sandra Dassenko, and James Cook. "Soy Protein, Phytate, and Iron Absorption in Humans." *American Journal of Clinical Nutrition,*

Volume 56, 1992: 573–578.

Hurrell, Richard, Manju Reddy, and James Cook. "Inhibition of Non-Haem Iron Absorption in Man by Polyphenolic-Containing Beverages." *British Journal of Nutrition, Volume 81*, 1999: 289–295.

Hyman, Dr. Mark. "Is Hidden *Fungus* Making You Ill?" Dr. Mark Hyman's website. drhyman.com/is-hidden-fungus-making-you-ill-1737/.

Ilardi, PhD, Stephen. "Dietary Sugar and Mental Illness: A Surprising Link" in *The Depression Cure. Psychology Today* website. www.psychologytoday.com/blog/the-depression-cure/200907/dietary-sugar-and-mental-illness-surprising-link.

"Inside Information on Important Innovations in Bio-Science and Technology: Liquid 'Stabilized Oxygen.'" *Bio/Tech News*, 2000. www.biotechnews.com/docs/vit-o_prn.html.

Ismail, Baraem, Bradley L. Reuhs, and S. Suzanne Nielsen. "Analysis of Food Contaminants, Residues, and Chemical Constituents of Concern." Seventeenth Report of the Joint FAO/WHO Expert Committee on Food Additives, World Health Organization techn. Rep. Ser. 1974, No. 539; FAO Nutrition Meetings Report Series, 1974, No. 53. World Health Organization, Geneva, 1974. The evaluations contained in this publication were prepared by the Joint FAO/WHO Expert Committee on Food Additives, which met in Geneva, June 25–July 4, 1973.

Jensen, DC, ND, PhD, Dr. Bernard. *Dr. Jensen's Guide to Better Bowel Care: A Complete Program for Tissue Cleansing through Bowel Management* (Avery, 1998).

——. *Health Magic Through Chlorophyll from Living Plant Life* (Bi World Industries, Inc.).

——. *Tissue Cleansing Through Bowel Management* (Escondido, Calif.: self-published, 1980).

Katch, Frank I. *History Makers.* www.sportsci.org/news/history/chittenden/chittenden.html.

"Kombucha Health Benefits." Written by "Kristen M." Food Renegade website. www.foodrenegade.com/kombucha-health-benefits/.

"Kombucha Tea." Mayo Clinic website. www.mayoclinic.com/health/

kombucha-tea/AN01658.

Kujovich, Jody. "Which Foods Keep the Body From Absorbing Iron from Pills?" Livestrong website. www.livestrong.com/article/280321-which-foods-keep-the-body-from-absorbing-iron-from-iron-pills/.

Leson, Gero, and Petra Pless. *Hemp Foods and Oils for Health* (Sebastopol, Calif.: Hemptech, 1991).

Mangels, PhD, RD, Reed. "Protein in the Vegan Diet." Vegetarian Resource Group website. VRG.org.

Manning, Richard. "The Oil We Eat: Following the Food Chain Back to Iraq." *Harper's*, February 2004.

Martin, Jeanne Marie, and Zoltan P. Rona, MD. *Complete Candida Yeast Guidebook, Everything You Need to Know About Prevention, Treatment & Diet, Revised Edition* (Prima Health, 2000).

Mayo Clinic website. www.mayoclinic.com.

McDougall, MD, John. "Nutrition in the Medical Clinic Part III" lecture. "Plant-Based Nutrition." eCornell University.

McMahon, James P. "Which Bottled Water Is the Best?" Sweetwater LLC website. www.cleanairpurewater.com/best_bottled_water.html.

Mercola, Dr. Joseph. "Everything You HAVE TO KNOW about Dangerous Genetically Modified Foods." Dr. Joseph Mercola's website. October 17, 2009. articles.mercola.com/sites/articles/archive/2009/10/17/everything-you-have-to-know-about-dangerous-genetically-modified-foods.aspx.

——. "Here's the Smarter Oil Alternative I Recommend to Replace Those Other Oils in Your Kitchen." Dr. Joseph Mercola's website. products.mercola.com/coconut-oil/.

——. "Juicing: Your Key to Radiant Health." Dr. Joseph Mercola's website. juicing.mercola.com/sites/juicing/juicing.aspx.

——. "Learn the Truth About Soy: Just How Much Soy Do Asians Eat?" Dr. Joseph Mercola's website. January 9, 2000. articles.mercola.com/sites/articles/archive/2000/01/09/truth-about-soy.aspx.

——. "More Scientific Support for Using Olive Oil." Dr. Joseph Mercola's website. articles.mercola.com/sites/articles/archive/2005/01/29/olive-oil-part-three.aspx.

——. "The Negative Health Effects of Chlorine." Dr. Joseph Mercola's website. February 28, 2001. articles.mercola.com/sites/articles/newsletter-archive/2001/.../28.aspx.

——. "Slathering on Sunscreen Does Not Prevent Cancer." Dr. Joseph Mercola's website. articles.mercola.com/sites/articles/archive/2003/08/02/sunscreen-cancer.aspx.

——. "Tap Water Toxins: Is Your Water Trying to Kill You?" Dr. Joseph Mercola's website. February 7, 2009. articles.mercola.com/sites/articles/archive/2001/01/07/chlorinated-water2.aspx.

——. "Vitamin B12: Are You Getting It?" Dr. Mercola's website. January 30, 2002. www.mercola.com/2002/jan/30/vitamin_b12.htm.

National Institutes of Health website. February 17, 2009. nccam.nih.gov/health/probiotics/D345.pdf.

Natural Health School website. www.naturalhealthschool.com/acid-alkaline.html.

"Natural Secret to Heal Most Health Problems Revealed to US Public." *Vegetarian Times,* February 2001.

Nature.org website. www.nature.org/ourinitiatives/urgentissues/rainforests/rainforests-facts.xml.

Navratilova, Martina. "Eat the Right Kinds of Protein: Don't Overdo Protein; Do it Right. Here's How." *AARP,* May 22, 2009.

Nazor, Nina. "All About Insulin." People and Diabetes website. peopleanddiabetes.com/id26.html.

Nielsen, Forrest. "Do You Have Trouble Sleeping? More Magnesium Might Help." USDA's Agricultural Research Service website. www.ars.usda.gov/News/docs.htm?docid=15617&pf=1&cg_id=0.

"Not Such Sweet News About Agave." *Berkeley Wellness Alert,* December 17, 2010. www.berkeleywellnessalerts.com/alerts/healthy_eating/Agave-Versus-Refined-Sugar211-1.html.

"Nutrition of Sprouting Seeds." Livestrong website. www.livestrong.com/article/288551-nutrition-of-sprouting-seeds/#ixzz1AZqr74pP.

O'Connor, Anahad. "The Claim: Cinnamon Oil Kills Bacteria." *New York Times,* September 7, 2009. www.nytimes.com/2009/09/08/

health/08real.html.

The Office of Dietary Supplements of the US Government website. nccam.nih.gov/health/supplements/wiseuse.htm.

Ogden, Lillie. "The Environmental Impact of a Meat-Based Diet." *Vegetarian Times,* February 2001. www.vegetariantimes.com/features/ft_eco_living/574.

Ott, John. *Light, Radiation and You: How to Stay Healthy* (Devin-Adair Publishers, 1982).

Pearson, Owen. "Vegetarian Foods Containing the B-5 Vitamin." Livestrong website. www.livestrong.com/article/339181-vegetarian-foods-containing-the-b-5-vitamin/#ixzz1SYBEgBD2.

Pereira, M.A. and V.L., Fulgoni, 3rd. "Consumption of 100% Fruit Juice and Risk of Obesity and Matabolic Syndrome: Findings from the National Health and Nutrition Examination Survey 1999–2004." *Journal of the American College of Nutrition. 29(6),* December 2010:625–9.

"Phytoestrogens and Breast Cancer—Fact Sheet #01." Revised July 2001. Cornell University website. envirocancer.cornell.edu/factsheet/diet/fs1.phyto.cfm.

Pitchford, Paul. *Healing With Whole Foods* (North Atlantic Books, 2002).

Popke, Michael. "Studies Reveal More Chlorine Risks, Including Cancer." Athletic Business website. September 14, 2010. athleticbusiness.com/editors/blog/default.aspx?id=236.

Pottenger, Francis Marion. *Pottenger's Cats: A Study in Nutrition by Francis Marion Pottenger* (Price-Pottenger Nutrition Foundation, June 1, 1995).

"Probiotic Identified to Treat Ulcers (Counters H. pylori)." American Society for Microbiology. February 24, 2011. Free Republic website. www.freerepublic.com/focus/f-chat/2679352/posts.

"Professionals Urge End to Water Fluoridation." NewsLI website. November 25, 2007. www.newsli.com/2007/11/25/professionals-urge-end-to-water-fluoridation/.

Raloff, Janet. "Vitamin D Boosts Calcium Potency." *Science News* website. www.sciencenews.org/view/generic/id/6775/title/Food_

for_Thought_Vitamin_D_Boosts_Calcium_Potency.

Regan, Tom. *The Case for Animal Rights* (University of California Press, 1983).

Robbins, John. "Diet for a New America." Veg Source website. www.vegsource.com/news/2009/09/how-to-win-an-argument-with-a-meat-eater.html.

——. "2,500 Gallons All Wet?" Earthsave website. www.earthsave.org/environment/water.htm.

Rose, Natalia. *The Raw Food Diet Detox* (HarperCollins Publishers, 2006)

Rutz, Jim. "The Trouble with Soy." WorldNetDaily website. 2010. www.wnd.com/news/article.asp?ARTICLE_ID=53327.

Sandy Simmons's Connective Tissue Disorder website. www.ctds.info/index.html.

Schlosser, Eric. *Fast Food Nation: The Dark Side of the American Meal* (New York: HarperCollins, 2002).

"School Drinking Water Unsafe: Schools in All 50 States, Especially Those with Private Supplies, Contain High Levels of Toxins." CBSNews—Healthwatch website. September 25, 2009. www.cbsnews.com/stories/2009/09/25/health/main5338720.shtml?source=related_story

Sheegan, Daniel M., and Daniel R. Doerge. Letter to Dockets Management Branch (HFA-305). February 18, 1999. The letter was posted on the abcnews.com website as "Scientists Protest Soy Approval."

Shomon, Mary. "The Controversy over Soy and Thyroid Health." About.com website. May 27, 2009. thyroid.about.com/cs/soyinfo/a/soy_3.htm.

Simontacchi, C. *The Crazy Makers: How the Food Industry Is Destroying Our Brains and Harming Our Children* (Penguin, 2008).

Singer, Peter. *Practical Ethics* (Cambridge University Press, 1999).

Sircus, Dr. Mark. "Diabetes—Acid Conditions and Treatment with Sodium Bicarbonate." New Paradigms of Diabetic Care website. diabetic.imva.info/index.php/treatments/diabetes-acid-conditions-

and-treatment-with-sodium-bicarbonate/.

——. "The Secrets of Light: Cancer and the Sun." *Nourished Magazine,* December 2008. nourishedmagazine.com.au/blog/articles/the-secrets-of-light-cancer-and-the-sun.

Smith, Derek. "What Are the Benefits of Calcium Bentonite Clay?" Livestrong website. www.livestrong.com/article/201565-what-are-the-benefits-of-calcium-bentonite-clay/#ixzz1N7bf1183.

Staciokas, Linden. "Growing Sprouts Is Easy, Nutritious Way to Satisfy Veggie Cravings." For the *Fairbanks Daily News-Miner,* April 20, 2010. www.newsminer.com/view/full_story/7148528/article-Growing-sprouts-is-easy--nutritious-way-to-satisfy-veggie-cravings-.

Sterling, Joseph. "Secrets of Robust Health" newsletter. Healing Waters website. www.healingwatersforhealth.com/GetAttachment.pdf.

"Stevia." Tufts University Medical Center website. www.tuftsmedicalcenter.org/apps/Healthgate/Article.aspx?chunkiid=21876.

Stillwell, Sophie. "Vegetarian Sources of B Vitamins." Livestrong website. www.livestrong.com/article/208601-vegetarian-sources-of-b-vitamins/#ixzz1SYDIiRlw.

"Summary of NRDC'S Test Results: Bottled Water Contaminants Found." Natural Resources Defense Council website. www.nrdc.org/water/drinking/bw/appa/asp.

"Sunscreens Exposed: 9 Surprising Truths. EWG's Skin Deep—Sunscreens 2011." Environmental Working Group website. June 23, 2011. breakingnews.ewg.org/2011sunscreen/sunscreens-exposed/sunscreens-exposed-9-surprising-truths/.

Tabak, Alan J. "Magnesium-Rich Foods Reduce Diabetes Risk, Study Says." *Harvard Crimson,* January 21, 2004.

Tuntipopipat, Siriporn, Kunchit Judprasong, Christophe Zedet, Emorn Wasantwisut, Pattanee Winichagoon, Somsri Charoenkiatkul, Richard Hurrell, and Thomas Walczyk. "Chili, but Not Turmeric, Inhibits Iron Absorption in Young Women from an Iron-Fortified Composite Meal." *The Journal of Nutrition, Volume 136,* 2006: 2970–2974.

Walsh, RD, Stephen. "Vegan Society B12 Factsheet." Vegan Society website. www.vegansociety.com/lifestyle/nutrition/b12.aspx.

Weigel, Jen. "Healthy Eating with a Spiritual Twist." Chicago Now website. July 20, 2009. www.chicagonow.com/blogs/spiritual-dammit/2009/07/healthy-eating-with-a-spiritual-twist.html#ixzz1S8wMYSoL.

Dr. Andrew Weil's website. www.drweil.com.

"What We Eat in America, NHANES 2001–2002, 1 Day, Individuals 1+ Years, Excluding Breast-Fed Children and Pregnant or Lactating Females." Agricultural Research Service website. www.ars.usda.gov/SP2UserFiles/Place/12355000/pdf/0102/usualintaketables2001-02.pdf.

"Where Exactly Does Vitamin B12 Come From?" The Vegan Forum website. www.veganforum.com/forums/archive/index.php/t-6856.ht.

White, Scott. "The Benefits of Glutamine Supplements." Article 2008 website. article2008.com/Art/60332/561/The-Benefits-of-Glutamine-Supplements.html.

Wigmore, Ann, and the Hippocrates Health Institute, Inc. *The Wheatgrass Book: How to Grow and Use Wheatgrass to Maximize Your Health and Vitality* (Avery Health Guides, 1985).

Wilens, T.E., J. Biederman, T.J. Spencer, J. Frazier, J. Prince, J. Bostic, M. Rater, J. Soriano, M. Hatch, M. Sienna, RB Millstein, and A. Abrantes. "Controlled Trial of High Doses of Pemoline for Adults with Attention-Deficit/Hyperactivity Disorder." *Journal of Clinical Psychopharmacology,* June 1999, 19(3):257–64.

Wilson, Dr. Lawrence. "Vitamin D Update 2010." Dr. Lawrence Wilson's website. www.drlwilson.com/ARTICLES/VITAMIN%20D.htm.

Yerba Prima website. www.yerba prima.com.

Young, PhD, Robert O., and Shelley Redford. *The Ph Miracle for Weight Loss* (New York and Boston: Warner Wellness, 2006).

Endnotes

1 "Doing it on Your Own: Eating Vegetarian." McGill University website. June 30, 2010. www.mcgill.ca/fitatmcgill/nutrition/doingit/veg/.

2 Excerpt from the book's order form. See www.nutrientrich.com/1/prevent-and-reverse-heart-disease.html.

3 McDougall, MD, John. "Nutrition in the Medical Clinic Part III" lecture. "Plant-Based Nutrition." eCornell University.

4 Campbell, T. Colin. "Principles of Nutritional Health." "Plant-Based Nutrition,. eCornell University, and the T. Colin Campbell Foundation. 2010.

5 Ibid.

6 Regan, Tom. *The Case for Animal Rights.* University of California Press, 1983.

7 Francione, Gary, and Robert Garner. *The Animal Rights Debate: Abolition or Regulation.* Columbia University Press, 2010.

8 Singer, Peter. *Practical Ethics.* Cambridge University Press, 1999.

9 Robbins, John. "2,500 Gallons All Wet?" Earthsave website. www.earthsave.org/environment/water.htm.

10 Ibid.

11 "Mission 2012: Clean Water." Massachusetts Institute of Technology (MIT) website. web.mit.edu/12.000/www/m2012/finalwebsite/problem/agriculture.shtml.

12 "U.S. Could Feed 800 Million People with Grain that Livestock Eat, Cornell Ecologist Advises Animal Scientist; Future Water and Energy Shortages Predicted to Change Face of American Agriculture." *Cornell University Science News,* August 7, 1997.

13 Manning, Richard. "The Oil We Eat: Following the Food Chain Back to Iraq." *Harper's,* February 2004.

14 Pimentel, David, and Marcia Pimentel. "Sustainability of Meat-Based and Plant-Based Diets and the Environment."[1,2,3] *The American Journal of Clinical Nutrition, vol. 78, no. 3,* 6605–35, September 2003. www.ajcn.org/content/78/3/660S.full. [1 From the Department of Ecology and Evolutionary Biology, Cornell University, Ithaca, NY; 2 Presented at the Fourth International Congress on Vegetarian Nutrition, held in Loma Linda, CA, April 8–11, 2002.

Published proceedings edited by Joan Sabaté and Sujatha Rajaram, Loma Linda University, Loma Linda, CA; 3 Address reprint requests to D Pimentel, Department of Ecology and Evolutionary Biology, Cornell University, 5126 Comstock Hall, Ithaca, NY 14853. E-mail: dp18@cornell.edu.]

15 Nature.org website. www.nature.org/ourinitiatives/urgentissues/rainforests/rainforests-facts.xml.

16 "Food from the Rainforests." Rainforest Action Network website. ran.org/fileadmin/materials/education/factsheets/RAN_Rainforest Food.pdf.

17 Ogden, Lillie. "The Environmental Impact of a Meat-Based Diet." *Vegetarian Times* magazine. www.vegetariantimes.com/features/ft_eco_living/574.

18 Ibid.

19 Ibid.

20 Robbins, John. *Diet for a New America.* Veg Source website. www.vegsource.com/news/2009/09/how-to-win-an-argument-with-a-meat-eater.html.

21 "Hunger." FAO news release, September 14, 2010. UN website. www.wfp.org/hunger/stats,%20FAO%20news%20release,%2014%20September%202010%20%20source.

22 "Average Mineral Content in Selected Vegetables, 1914–1997." Nutrition Security Institute website. www.nutritionsecurity.org/PDF/Mineral%20Content%20in%20Vegetables.pdf. This United States Department of Agriculture source was listed at the bottom of the chart: Lindlahr, 1914, Hamaker, 1982, US Department of Agriculture, 1963 and 1997.

23 "Eighty Year Decline in Mineral Content of Medium Apple." Nutrition Security Institute website. www.nutritionsecurity.org/PDF/Mineral%20Content%20of%20One%20Apple.pdf. This United States Department of Agriculture source was listed at the bottom of the chart: Lindlahr, 1914, Hamaker, 1982, US Department of Agriculture, 1963 and 1997.

24 "Dietary Supplement Fact Sheet: Calcium." US Office of Diet Supplements, National Institutes of Health website. ods.od.nih.gov/factsheets/Calcium-QuickFacts/.

25 "Doing it on Your Own: Eating Vegetarian." McGill University website. June 30, 2010. www.mcgill.ca/fitatmcgill/nutrition/doingit/veg/.

26 Bassler, Dr. Anthony. "A Common Mistake that Prevents Most People from Losing Weight…and How to Avoid It! Why This Simple 'First Step' Should Be Part of Any Weight Management, Anti-Aging and Health Improvement Program." *Vegetarian Times,* January 2004.

27 Baroody, Dr. Theodore. *Alkalize or Die.* Holographic Health Inc., December 1991.

28 "PH Balance." Lesson 18. The Natural Health School website. www.naturalhealthschool.com/pH-balance.html.

29 Young, PhD, Robert O., and Shelley Redford Young. *The pH Miracle for Weight Loss.* New York and Boston: Warner Wellness, 2006.

30 "The Cause of Disease, PH Balance, acid and Alkaline Imbalance." Natural Health School website. www.naturalhealthschool.com/acid-alkaline.html.

31 Jensen, Dr. Bernard. *Tissue Cleansing Through Bowel Management.* Escondido, Calif.: Self-published, 1980.

32 Anderson, ND, NMD, Dr. Richard. "Colon Plaque—Mucoid Plaque." Cleanse.net website. cleanse.net/mucoidplaque-2.aspx. Dr. Richard Anderson, ND, NMD, is the author of *Cleanse and Purify Yourself* (Avery Trade, revised edition 1998).

33 Kalenite pill product website. www.yerba.com/storefront/item.asp?id=80.

34 "The Arbor, Alcohol and Drug and Rehab." Detoxnet website. www.detox.net.au/articles/detoxification.html.

35 Ibid.

36 "'Healing Clays' Hold Promise in Fight Against MRSA Superbug Infections and Disease." Arizona State University—Biodesign Institute website. April 7, 2008. www.biodesign.asu.edu.

37 El, Dr. Akilah M. "The Health Benefits of Bentonite Clay." Dr. Akilah El's website: The Natural Health and Holistic World According to Dr. Akilah El." docakilah.wordpress.com/2011/06/09/the-health-benefits-of-bentonite-clay/.

38 Pickut, Walt. "What Are the Benefits of Calcium Bentonite Clay?"

Livestrong website. www.livestrong.com/article/201565-what-are-the-benefits-of-calcium-bentonite-clay/#ixzz1XBmLOTRQ.

39 Jensen, Dr. Bernard. *Dr. Jensen's Guide to Better Bowel Care: A Complete Program for Tissue Cleansing through Bowel Management.* Avery, 1998.

40 Ibid.

41 Sterling, Joseph. *Secrets of Robust Health* newsletter, Vol. 5, No. 1, March 2004. www.healingwatersforhealth.com/GetAttachment.pdf.

42 Howell, Dr. E. *Enzyme Nutrition.* Avery Publishing Group Inc., 1985.

43 Cheung, FRCP, Dr. Anthony. "Enzymes." Enerex website. www.enerex.ca/en/articles/digestive-enzymes.

44 Howell, *Enzyme Nutrition.*

45 Ibid.

46 Cheung, "Enzymes."

47 Ibid.

48 Azulay, Sol. "There's More to Sprouts than Just a Little Crunch in Your Salad." Interview with the *San Diego Earth Times.* November 1997.

49 Ibid.

50 Ibid.

51 "Olive Oil Acid 'Cuts Cancer Risk.'" BBC News website. January 10, 2005. news.bbc.co.uk/go/pr/fr/-/2/hi/health/4154269.stm.

52 "Mercola, Dr. Joseph "Here's the Smarter Oil Alternative I Recommend to Replace Those Other Oils in Your Kitchen." Dr. Joseph Mercola's website. products.mercola.com/coconut-oil/.

53 Ibid.

54 Johnson, Lorie. "Coconut Oil Tauted as Alzheimers Remedy" Lorie Johnson CBN News Medical Reporter, Jan. 05, 2012, The Christian Broadcasting Network website, www.cbn.com/cbnnews/health-science/2012/January/Coconut-Oil-Touted-as-Alzheimers-Remedy/.

55 Weigel, Jen. "Healthy Eating with a Spiritual Twist." *Chicago Now* website. July 20, 2009. www.chicagonow.com/blogs/

spiritual-dammit/2009/07/healthy-eating-with-a-spiritual-twist.html#ixzz1S8wMYSoL.

56 Ibid.

57 Ibid.

58 Mercola, Dr. Joseph. "More Scientific Support for Using Olive Oil. Dr. Joseph Mercola's website. articles.mercola.com/sites/articles/archive/2005/01/29/olive-oil-part-three.aspx.

59 Ibid.

60 Coates, Dr. Wayne. "Chia History." Dr. Wayne Coates's website. www.azchia.com/chia_history.htm.

61 Cromie, William. "Genetic Secrets of Killer Fungus Found." *Harvard Gazette*. October 30, 1997. news.harvard.edu/gazette/1997/10.30/GeneticSecretso.html.

62 Hyman, Dr. Mark. "Is Hidden *Fungus* Making You Ill?" Dr. Mark Hyman's website. drhyman.com/is-hidden-fungus-making-you-ill-1737/.

63 Ibid.

64 Ibid.

65 Ibid.

66 Brock, Dr. Rovenia. Interview with Bob Green on foods that help relieve stress. Oprah Radio. January 1, 2008.

67 White, Scott. "The Benefits of Glutamine Supplements." Personal Power Training website. www.personalpowertraining.net/Articles/glutamine_benefits.htm.

68 Cohen, Bryan. "Natural Cures for Enlarged Thyroid." eHow website. www.ehow.com/way_5317305_natural-cures-enlarged-thyroid.html#ixzz1SYtyAarn.

69 "Dietary Supplement Fact Sheet: Iron." US Office of Dietary Supplements, National Institutes of Health website. ods.od.nih.gov/factsheets/iron/.

70 Ibid.

71 "What We Eat in America, NHANES 2001–2002, 1 day, Individuals 1+ Years, Excluding Breast-Fed Children and Pregnant or Lactating

Females." The US Department of Agriculture, Agricultural Research Service website. September 2005. www.ars.usda.gov/SP2UserFiles/Place/12355000/pdf/0102/usualintaketables2001-02.pdf.

72 Nielsen, Forrest. "Trouble Sleeping? More Magnesium Might Help." The US Department of Agriculture, Agricultural Research Service website. www.ars.usda.gov/News/docs.htm?docid=15617&pf=1&cg_id=0.

73 Ibid.

74 "Probiotic Identified to Treat Ulcers." *Science News* website. February 24, 2011. www.sciencedaily.com/releases/2011/02/110224121905.htm.

75 "An Introduction to Probiotics." National Institutes of Health website. February 17, 2009. nccam.nih.gov/health/probiotics/D345.pdf.

76 McDougall, "Nutrition in the Medical Clinic."

77 Katch, Frank I. *History Makers.* Sportscience.org website. www.sportsci.org/news/history/chittenden/chittenden.html.

78 McDougall, Dr. John. "A Brief History of Protein, Passion, Social Bigotry, Rats and Enlightenment." *The McDougall Newsletter, Volume 2, Number 12.* December 2003. www.nealhendrickson.com/mcdougall/031200puprotein.htm.

79 D'Adamo, Dr. Peter J., with Catherine Whitney. *Eat Right 4 Your Type.* "Blood Type O, Food, Beverage and Supplement List." New York: The Berkley Publishing Group, 2000.

80 Ibid.

81 Mangels, PhD, RD, Reed. "Protein in the Vegan Diet." Vegetarian Resource Group website. www.vrg.org/nutrition/protein.htm.

82 Navratilova, Martina. "Eat the Right Kinds of Protein: Don't Overdo Protein; Do it Right. Here's How." *AARP.* May 22, 2009.

83 McDougall, "A Brief History."

84 The Cleveland Clinic website. my.clevelandclinic.org/p2/us_news_rankings.

85 "Women's Cardiovascular Center." The Cleveland Clinic website. my.clevelendclinic.org/heart/women/nutritioncorner_vegetarian.aspx.

86 From the question and answer library on Dr. Andrew Weil's website. Published December 11, 2002; updated March 21, 2005. www.drweil.com/drw/u/id/QAA142995.

87 Ibid.

88 Gordon, MEd, RD, Dennis. "Vegetable Proteins Can Stand Alone." *Journal of the American Dietetic Association, volume 96, issue 3.* March 1996.

89 Mangels, "Protein." The website also contains some menus and protein guidelines.

90 Information about hemp seeds comes from Gero Leson and Petra Pless's "Hemp Foods and Oils for Health." Hemptech, Sebastopol, California. Gero Leson, DEnv (www.drbronner.com/pdf/hemp-nutrition.pdf), is an environmental scientist and consultant with extensive experience in food and fiber uses of hemp and other renewable resources.

91 "Alert: Protein Drinks: You Don't Need the Extra Protein or the Heavy Metals Our Tests Found." *Consumer Reports* website. www.consumerreports.org/cro/magazine-archive/2010/july/food/protein-drinks/overview/index.htm.

92 This quote is taken from an article ("Dangers of Whey Protein" by Chris Deoudes) in the *Livestrong* newsletter. Article reviewed by Roman Tsivkin. June 15, 2011. www.livestrong.com/article/217799-the-dangers-of-whey-protein/#ixzz1AYahdybh.

93 Ibid.

94 Damato, Dr. Gregory. "GM-Soy: Destroy the Earth and Humans for Profit." Natural News website. May 27, 2009. www.naturalnews.com/026334_soy_Roundup_GMO.html#ixzz1RzIZAWwh.

95 Fallon, Sallon, and Mary G. Enig, PhD. "Soy's Dark Side: Newest Research on Why You Should Avoid Soy." DC Nutrition website. www.dcnutrition.com/news/Detail.CFM?RecordNumber=480.

96 Damato, "GM-Soy."

97 Ibid.

98 Mercola, Dr. Joseph. "Learn the Truth About Soy: Just How Much Soy Do Asians Eat?" Dr. Mercola's website. January 9, 2000. articles.mercola.com/sites/articles/archive/2000/01/09/truth-about-soy.aspx.

99 Fallon and Enig, "Soy's Dark Side."

100 Bellatti, Andy. "You Ask, I Answer: Soy Portein Isolate." Medpedia.com website. April 16, 2011. www.medpedia.com/news_analysis/98-Small-Bites/entries/71677-You-Ask-I-Answer-Soy-Protein-Isolate.

101 Rutz, Jim. "The Trouble with Soy." World Net Daily website. www.wnd.com/news/article.asp?ARTICLE_ID=53327. 2010. This article was originally titled "Soy Is Making Kids 'Gay,'" but after a huge backlash he re-titled it "The Trouble with Soy."

102 Sheegan, Daniel M., and Daniel R. Doerge. Letter to Dockets Management Branch (HFA-305). February 18, 1999. The letter was posted on the abcnews.com website as "Scientists Protest Soy Approval."

103 Bellatti. "You Ask."

104 Cousens MD, Gabriel, and David Rainoshek. *There Is a Cure for Diabetes*. Berkeley, Calif.: North Atlantic Books, 2008.

105 Ibid.

106 Rutz, "The Trouble with Soy."

107 "Agriculture Fact Book 98." US Department of Agriculture website. www.usda.gov/news/pubs/fbook98/ch1a.htm.

108 "High-Fructose Corn Syrup: Everything You Wanted to Know, but Were Afraid to Ask." *American Journal of Clinical Nutrition,* 88(6):1715S. December 2008.

109 Pereira, M.A., and V.L. Fulgoni 3rd. "Consumption of 100% Fruit Juice and Risk of Obesity and Metabolic Syndrome: Findings from the National Health and Nutrition Examination Survey 1999-2004." *Journal of the American College of Nutrition 29(6)*: 625–9. December 2010. Abstract available at www.ncbi.nlm.nih.gov/pubmed/21677126.

110 From the US National Library of Medicine, National Institutes of Health website. www.ncbi.nlm.nih.gov/pubmed/19064535. PMID: 19064535.

111 Ilardi, PhD, Stephen. "Dietary Sugar and Mental Illness: A Surprising Link" in *The Depression Cure. Psychology Today* website. www.psychologytoday.com/blog/the-depression-cure/200907/dietary-sugar-and-mental-illness-surprising-link.

112 Goulart, Frances Sheridan. "Are You Sugar Smart? Linked to Heart Attacks, Kidney Disease, Diabetes and Other Diseases, Sugar is to the '90s What Cholesterol Was to the '80s—Includes 9 Ways to Cope with Sugar Cravings." *American Fitness.* March–April 1991. findarticles.com/p/articles/mi_m0675/is_n2_v9/ai_10722552/.

113 Ibid.

114 Ibid.

115 "Not Such Sweet News About Agave." *Berkeley Wellness Alerts.* December 17, 2010. www.berkeleywellnessalerts.com/alerts/healthy_eating/Agave-Versus-Refined-Sugar211-1.html?zkDo=emailArticlePrompt.

116 Ibid.

117 "Cinnamon and Honey." *Weekly World News.* January 17, 1995.

118 Gittleman, PhD, CNS, Ann Louise, *Get the Sugar Out.* New York: Three Rivers Press, 1996, p. 15.

119 "Stevia." Tufts University Medical Center website. www.tuftsmedical center.org/apps/Healthgate/Article.aspx?chunkiid=21876.

120 Ibid.

121 Ibid.

122 "Find a Vitamin or Supplement: Stevia." WebMD website. www.webmd.com/vitamins-supplements/ingredientmono-682-STEVIA.aspx?activeIngredientId=682&activeIngredientName=STEVIA.

123 The information from this section comes from Fran Gare's *The Sweet Miracle of Xylitol* (Basic Health Publications, Inc., 2003).

124 Edwards, Michael. "Healthy Sugar Alternatives: Understanding Both Healthy & Not So Healthy Sugars with Their Glycemic Index." *Organic Lifestyle* magazine, June 12, 2009. www.organiclife stylemagazine.com/blog/healthy-sugar-alternatives.php. This is a good source for the glycemic index of various sugars.

125 Pearson, Owen. "Vegetarian Foods Containing the B-5 Vitamin." Livestrong website. www.livestrong.com/article/339181-vegetarian-foods-containing-the-b-5-vitamin/#ixzz1SYBEgBD2.

126 Kresser L. AC, Chris "The Little Known (but Crucial) Difference Between Folate and Folic Acid" Chris Kessler, LAc website. March 9, 2012 chriskresser.com/folate-vs-folic-acid.

127 Mercola, Dr. Joseph. "Vitamin B12: Are Your Getting It?" Dr. Mercola's website. www.mercola.com/2002/jan/30/vitamin_b12.htm.

128 "Where Exactly Does Vitamin D Come From?" Vegan Forum website. www.veganforum.com/forums/showthread.php?6856-Where-exactly-does-Vitamin-B12-come-from&s=944287d5025a9e833aa9bb763923fdbb.

129 Walsh, RD, Stephen. "Vegan Society B12 Factsheet." Vegan Society website. www.vegansociety.com/lifestyle/nutrition/b12.aspx.

130 Goulart, "Are You Sugar Smart?"

131 Mercola, Dr. Joseph. "Vitamin D Update 2010." Dr. Lawrence Wilson's website. www.drlwilson.com/ARTICLES/VITAMIN%20D.htm.

132 Ibid.

133 Mercola, Dr. Joseph. "Why the New Vitamin D Recommendations Spell Disaster for Your Health." Dr. Mercola's newsletter, December 11, 2010. Dr. Mercola's website. articles.mercola.com/sites/articles/archive/2010/12/11/vitamin-d-update-carole-baggerly-and-dr-cannell.aspx.

134 Raloff, Janet. "Vitamin D Boosts Calcium Potency." *Science News* website. www.sciencenews.org/view/generic/id/6775/title/Food_for_Thought_Vitamin_D_Boosts_Calcium_Potency.

135 Hattersley, Joseph G. "The Negative Health Effects of Chlorine." Available at findarticles.com/p/articles/mi_m0ISW/is_2003_May/ai_100767859/ or on Dr. Mercola's website at www.mercola.com/Downloads/bonus/chlorine/default.aspx?s_kwcid=TC|15735|chlorine||S|b|9483696664&gclid=CMjlxLKX6qwCFciC5Qod8y75Nw.

136 Popke, Michael. "Studies Reveal More Chlorine Risks, Including Cancer." Athletic Business website. September 14, 2010. athleticbusiness.com/editors/blog/default.aspx?id=236.

137 Connett, PhD, Paul. "50 Reasons to Oppose Fluoridation." St. Lawrence University (Canton, N.Y.). These "50 Reasons" were first compiled by Paul Connett and presented in person to the Fluoridation Forum in Ireland in October 2000. The document was refined in 2004 and published in *Medical Veritas*. See: www.fluoridealert.org/50reasons.htm. In the introduction to this 2004 version it was

explained that after over four years the Irish authorities had not been able to muster a response to the "50 Reasons," despite agreeing to do so in 2000.

137 Ibid.

138 Barclay, Eliza. "What's Best for Kids: Bottled Water or Fountains?" *National Geographic Daily News.* March 3, 1020. news.nationalgeographic.com/news/2010/02/100303-bottled-water-tap-schools/.

140 Associated Press. "Drinking Water at Schools Contains Lead, Pesticides, Other Toxins: Study." *New York Daily News.* September 25, 2009. articles.nydailynews.com/2009-09-25/entertainment/17930709_1_safe-drinking-water-act-water-supplies-five-schools/2.

141 "Bottled Water: Pure Drink or Pure Hype?" Natural Resources Defense Council website. www.nrdc.org/water/drinking/bw/bwinx.asp.

142 Ibid.

143 Masaru Emoto's website. www.masaru-emoto.net/english/e_ome_home.html.

144 Mercola, Dr. Joseph. "Juicing: Your Key to Radiant Health." Dr. Mercola's website. juicing.mercola.com/sites/juicing/juicing.aspx.

145 Wigmore, Ann, and the Hippocrates Health Institute, Inc. *The Wheatgrass Book: How to Grow and Use Wheatgrass to Maximize Your Health and Vitality.* Avery Health Guides, 1985.

146 Jensen, Dr. Bernard. *Health Magic Through Chlorophyll from Living Plant Life.* Jensen's Health and Nutrition, 1973.

147 Nazor, Nina. "All About Insulin." People and Diabetes website. peopleanddiabetes.com/id26.html.

148 Mercola, "Juicing."

149 Dyer, MS, RD, Diana. "What's in Kale? USDA Nutrient Content Data." 365 Days of Kale weblog. February 22, 2009. www.365daysofkale.com/2009/02/whats-in-kale-usda-nutrient-content.html.

150 Bolen, Jim. "Histamine/Anti-histamine and the Dangers of Taking Anti-histamine." Water Cure website. www.watercure2.org/histamines.htm.

151 Batmanghelidj, MD, Fereydoon. *ABC of Asthma, Allergies and Lupus, First Edition.* Global Health Solutions, Inc., 2000.

152 Pitchford, Paul, *Healing with Whole Foods, Third Edition*. Berkeley, Calif.: North Atlantic Books, 2002, pp. 224–5.

153 Ibid., p. 537.

154 Ibid., p. 545.

155 Ibid., p. 246.

156 O'Connor, Anahad. "The Claim: Cinnamon Oil Kills Bacteria." *New York Times*. September 7, 2009. www.nytimes.com/2009/09/08/health/08real.html.

157 "Honey and Cinnamon Cure." *Weekly World News*. January 17, 1995. weeklyworldnews.com/archive/.

158 "Kombucha Tea." Mayo Clinic website. www.mayoclinic.com/health/kombucha-tea/AN01658.

159 Mercola, Dr. Joseph. "Slathering on Sunscreen Does Not Prevent Cancer." Dr. Joseph Mercola's website. articles.mercola.com/sites/articles/archive/2003/08/02/sunscreen-cancer.aspx.

160 Douillard, DC, Dr. John. "Vitamin D: Astonishing Health Benefits." Dr. John Douillard's Lifespa.com website. www.lifespa.com/article.aspx?art_id=100&view=print.

161 Douillard, DC, Dr. John. "Sun Exposure: Don't Be Fooled By Your Sunscreen." Dr. John Douillard'sLifespa.com website. www.lifespa.com/article.aspx?art_id=114&view=print.

162 Douillard, "Vitamin D."

163 "Sunscreens Exposed: 9 Surprising Truths. EWG's Skin Deep—Sunscreens 2011." Environmental Working Group website. June 23, 2011. breakingnews.ewg.org/2011sunscreen/sunscreens-exposed/sunscreens-exposed-9-surprising-truths/.

164 Wigmore, *The Wheatgrass Book*.

165 Mercola, Dr. Joseph. "Everything You HAVE TO KNOW about Dangerous Genetically Modified Foods." Dr. Joseph Mercola's website. October 17, 2009. articles.mercola.com/sites/articles/archive/2009/10/17/everything-you-have-to-know-about-dangerous-genetically-modified-foods.aspx.

166 Staciokas, Linden. "Growing Sprouts Is Easy, Nutritious Way to Satisfy Veggie Cravings." *Fairbanks Daily News-Miner*. April 20, 2010.

www.newsminer.com/view/full_story/7148528/article-Growing-sprouts-is-easy--nutritious-way-to-satisfy-veggie-cravings-.

167 Azulay, Sol. International Specialty Supply website. www.sproutnet.com/sprouts_in_the_press.htm.

168 Phillips, John. "Conscious Gardening Workshop at Tree of Life." Tree of Life website. January 2009. www.treeoflife.nu/conscious gardening. AND "EM: Effective Microbial." EM Hawaii website. www.emhawaii.com/.

169 "Stabilized Oxygen." *Bio/Tech News*, 2000. www.biotechnews.com/docs/vit-o_prn.html.

170 "Code of Federal Regulations, Title 21, Volume 2." Revised as of April 1, 2009. US Government Printing Office, GPO Access CITE: 21CFR101.22. pp. 72–76.

171 Schlosser, Eric. *Fast Food Nation*. Perennial, an imprint of Harper Collins, 2001, 2002, p. 126.

172 Ibid.

173 "Consumer Group Calls for Ban on 'Flour Improver': Potassium Bromate Termed a Cancer Threat." Center for Science in the Public Interest website. July 19, 1999. www.cspinet.org/new/bromate.html.

174 Ibid.

175 Freedman, Rory, and Kim Barnouin. *Skinny Bitch*. Running Press, 2005, p. 58.

176 Kujovich, Jody. "Which Foods Keep the Body From Absorbing Iron from Pills?" Livestrong website. www.livestrong.com/article/280321-which-foods-keep-the-body-from-absorbing-iron-from-iron-pills/.

177 Freedman and Barnouin, *Skinny Bitch*.

178 Gray, Theodore. "A Change to Heat-Resistant Glass Has Had explosive Effects." PopSci website. April 26, 2011. www.popsci.com/science/article/2011-03/gray-matter-cant-take-heat.

179 McDougall, MD, John. "Alzheimer's Again Linked to Aluminum." Rense.com website. www.rense.comgeneral137/alum.htm.

180 Schaffer, Amanda. "Nervous About Nonstick? Easy to Clean and Incredibly Popular, This Cookware Is Still Considered Potentially

Toxic by Some Experts. *Good Housekeeping* Settles the Debate—and Tells You How to Use it Safely." *Good Housekeeping* website. www.goodhousekeeping.com/product-testing/reviews-tests/kitchen-cooking/nonstick-cookware-safety-facts.

181 Ibid.

182 Main, Emily. "This or That: Bleach vs. Vinegar to Kill Germs." Rodale website. www.rodale.com/natural-disinfectant?page=0%2C1.

Index

C

D

E

F

I

J

K

L

M

N

O

T

U

V

W

CPSIA information can be obtained
at www.ICGtesting.com
Printed in the USA
FSOW01n0024050515
6870FS